the**facts**

Post-traumatic Stress

thefacts

Post-traumatic Stress

SECOND EDITION

STEPHEN REGEL

Centre for Trauma, Resilience and Growth, Nottinghamshire
Healthcare NHS Foundation Trust and School of Education,
University of Nottingham, UK

STEPHEN JOSEPH

Centre for Trauma, Resilience and Growth, Nottinghamshire
Healthcare NHS Foundation Trust, and School of Education,
University of Nottingham, UK

OXFORD
UNIVERSITY PRESS

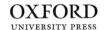

Great Clarendon Street, Oxford, OX2 6DP,
United Kingdom

Oxford University Press is a department of the University of Oxford.
It furthers the University's objective of excellence in research, scholarship,
and education by publishing worldwide. Oxford is a registered trade mark of
Oxford University Press in the UK and in certain other countries

First Edition published in 2010
Second Edition published in 2017

Impression: 1

Published in the United States of America by Oxford University Press
198 Madison Avenue, New York, NY 10016, United States of America

British Library Cataloguing in Publication Data

Data available

Library of Congress Control Number: 2016958445

ISBN 978–0–19–875811–2

Printed in Great Britain by
Clays Ltd, St Ives plc

SR: For Tina for her love and perseverance!
and Hannah and Tom as always.

SJ: For Vanessa

Foreword: Terry Waite

Since I wrote the forward to the first edition of this book, alas, the need for professional help to deal with the problem of traumatic stress has not diminished. Increasingly more and more members of the public are aware of this condition and recognize that it can be effectively treated. The recent attacks in Paris, Nice, Tunisia, Baghdad, and Brussels and elsewhere have had a profound psychological impact on many people, and this book will be of significant help to those involved in such tragedies.

Many years ago, when I jointly founded Hostage UK, we established a group of professionals who were willing to offer their help to former hostages and their families as and when required. This book, with its clear descriptions of the problem has played a major role in decreasing the resistance of many people who had little or no understanding of the condition but nevertheless suffered from it and sought our help. Not everyone who experiences a major traumatic incident in his or her life will suffer from the disorder. Again, this book, in a clear and concise way, presents the facts, and in so doing plays a major role in developing understanding of the condition, and enabling many to receive the help and support that they so urgently require.

Terry Waite CBE

Foreword: Atle Dyregrov

People all around the globe experience events that are potentially traumatic. Unfortunately, human-made and natural disasters are on the rise, together with accidents, suicide, murder, serious criminal acts, sexual assaults, and other extremely stressful events continue to affect the mental health of individuals, families, and society in general. Understanding trauma and its aftermath is not easy, especially when a person is in the midst of the resulting internal and external chaos. Trauma not only challenges our beliefs, it also disrupts the lives of individuals, families, and communities. This book offers both non-professionals and professionals a better understanding of the psychological impact of trauma, as well as offering ways to counteract and minimize the risk that such events present.

Trauma, in a simple way, can be divided into two types: complex trauma, usually the result of repetitive adverse childhood events, and single-event trauma, where there is one critical situation leading to after-reactions. Often there is a complex mix; people who experience a trauma have a history of previous losses or traumas that play a part in determining the resulting reactions. Regel and Joseph describe how pre-event, peri-event (happens during the event), and post-event factors can all determine people's responses. Disentangling the contributing factors is not easy to determine a cause of action when aiming to reduce untoward effects.

Their historical overview of our understanding of psychological trauma demonstrates how trauma has always been part of people's lives. Even after the introduction of post-traumatic stress disorder (PTSD) into psychiatry and psychology in 1980, the definition of what constitutes a trauma has been shifting over the years. Although the trauma 'breakthrough' in the professional field had strong military influence (from the Vietnam War), it has since then had a significant effect on our understanding of those who experience trauma in a civilian context. Actually, the loss of a family member is thought to be one of the events that accounts for the highest levels of PTSD. Recently, research within the medical field has also opened our eyes to the many individuals who develop post-traumatic stress in relation to experiences of Intensive Care treatment, stroke, and cancer, for example. The ever-broadening focus on trauma reactions now means that people can get help and support for reactions they formerly were left alone to cope with.

Heated debates over early intervention following trauma has clouded our vision in the trauma field. It should come as no surprise that it is especially difficult to prove that psychological interventions provided during the first days following exposure to a potentially traumatic event have the potential to reduce later trauma. It is difficult and may even be unethical to present affected individuals and families with research where questionnaires have to be filled out or research interviews conducted too close to the event. The early intervention debate has also been "poisoned" by the debate about psychological debriefing, based on studies that do not reflect how serious clinicians would work with affected individuals or groups. The debate following these studies caused a setback to the care and follow-up of people both directly and indirectly (first responders) affected by traumatic events. Fortunately, a new and more sober evaluation and discussion of these issues has, to some extent, 'rehabilitated' psychological debriefing and the use of early intervention. In this book, practical advice on how to intervene early reflects the authors' vast clinical and research knowledge in this area. This does not mean that therapy is indicated in most cases, but those rapid, timely, outreach initiatives that secure good individual, family, and community coping can be most effective when the world feels chaotic and dangerous.

Practical suggestions that can be used on various levels to support and assist both direct victims and emergency personnel exposed to extremely stressful events make the book very useful for those navigating new terrain following a traumatic event. The book explains and illustrates how the psychological impact from traumatic events can be handled and balanced by the knowledge that the same event can lead to growth, where one acknowledges strengths, prioritizes values, and regains a zest for life. The increased attention to the salutogenic consequences of trauma has infused the book with an optimistic tone.

Many books on trauma are available for sufferers and their families, and many are offered as 'self-help guides'. However, the vast majority of those exposed to traumatic events are far too avoidant to make use of the exercises. This book succeeds on two fronts, firstly it focuses on information to help individuals and families affected by traumatic events to understand and seek the appropriate support they need. Secondly, it will also greatly assist those responsible for providing that support with an understanding of the many nuances of how those affected by traumatic events are affected.

The practical format of the book, with its extensive use of case examples and suggestions, offers both those who have lived through a trauma and professional helpers many ways of understanding and coping with the trauma without becoming a superficial self-help guide.

Professor Atle Dyregrov
Center for Crisis Psychology and Department of Clinical Psychology,
Faculty of Psychology, University of Bergen, Norway

Preface

The range and diversity of the human response to extremely stressful and traumatic experiences is as extensive as the different traumatic events and stressors that confront human beings. From survivors of road-traffic collisions through to those who have experienced assault and rape, war veterans, survivors of disasters both human-made and natural, and the experience of refugees, trauma cuts across all human boundaries. Now, in the twenty-first century, there are new threats of global catastrophe (e.g. wars, terrorism, and ethnic and religious conflict). There are also the experiences of those who work in the emergency services, such as the police, fire and rescue services, health, and, of course, those who work for humanitarian agencies, who have to cope with trauma and human suffering often of staggering proportions.

This book is aimed at providing a map of the 'landscape' of trauma and its emotional aftermath. The reader is given the necessary information, guided directions, and helpful signposts in order to understand the key issues affecting the reactions of individuals, families, and communities exposed to traumatic events.

In our own ways, we have each been involved in the study, observation, research, counselling, and treatment of traumatized and bereaved individuals, families, communities, and those in the emergency services and military veterans, for over 30 years. We hope that this book will be helpful to people exposed to traumatic events and to their partners, friends, and families, who are themselves often in need of information. In the aftermath, confusion is common. Survivors may not understand what is happening to them. Families and friends may feel rejected and struggle to know how to help. We offer guidance and advice, some dos and don'ts, as well as directions for further support. For those who wish to know more, we end with suggestions for further reading and Internet resources.

We have also often been asked, when presenting seminars, lectures, and workshops, for an accessible introduction to trauma and post-traumatic stress. The secondary audience of this book is the professionals who come into contact with traumatized individuals on a daily basis—general practitioners, social workers, mental health nurses, mental health practitioners in primary and secondary care such as those in the Improving Access to Psychological Therapy service, counsellors, and health and social care professionals in training.

This book will also be a valuable and practical resource for those who work in high-risk professions (e.g. the emergency services; those involved in peer support for colleagues exposed to traumatic events in the workplace, including humanitarian aid workers who will find this an accessible introduction to the field).

Finally, we owe an enormous debt of gratitude to our many clients, patients, and participants in our research studies and clinical practice, who have taught us so much over the years and contributed their case studies contained in many of the chapters, which they have generously allowed us to share in order to illustrate and highlight their many diverse experiences. They know who they are, and we cannot thank them enough.

Stephen Regel
Stephen Joseph

Acknowledgements

Our thanks are still due to Liz Edwards who retired after many years of NHS service for her patience, forbearance, and help with the original edition and her excellent support over the years. We also express our gratitude to Caroline Smith and Nic Wilson of Oxford University Press for their invaluable advice, patience, and support throughout, and for keeping us in check and on course, and to Jenny Wright (OUP) who advised on the first edition.

We also wish to acknowledge the contribution of many colleagues to our thinking about our work over the years. They have not only been thoughtful, caring, and professional colleagues but also good, 'critical' friends who have played a huge part in our continuing enthusiasm and motivation to continue with this work, thank you.

SR wishes to thank Arlene Healey former head the Family Trauma Centre (FTC) in Belfast for her continued friendship, sound, pragmatic experience, and advice over the years, as well as the excellent, dedicated team at the FTC for making me feel part of the family; Dr Marion Gibson, a good friend and colleague, who gave me many opportunities over the years; Professor Peter Berliner from the University of Aarhus, for his warmth, enthusiasm, experience and for sharing his knowledge and experience about 'community' approaches to trauma; Dr Atle Dyregrov, Director, Centre for Crisis Psychology, Bergen for continuing to contribute so much to my thinking around early interventions for individuals, groups, and families following trauma and traumatic bereavement, many would do well to embrace his practical and creative approaches in the field; Dr Anne Hackmann at the Oxford Cognitive Therapy Centre for her insightful supervision in the past; Claire Hallam at Freeth Cartwright Solicitors for helpful comments on the section on litigation; and Dave Hannigan, Ali Rowlands, Tracey Reid, Sigiriya Aebischer-Perone, Roddy McNidder, Mark Woodland, Mark Lamerton, Lynne McDermott, Katie Dunn, and David Alexander for their unfailing support over the years.

Thanks are also due to the many students I have come into contact with over the years and who still continue to contribute significantly to the intellectual (and social!) life and development of the Centre for Trauma, Resilience and Growth (CTRG) in Nottingham—please don't ever stop being a challenge!

Last, but by no means least, thanks are due in no small measure to my friend, colleague, and co-author, Stephen Joseph, for not only keeping me on track but also broadening and challenging my thinking about my work in trauma.

SJ would like to thank his colleagues at the University of Nottingham for their support; the students of the Masters in Trauma Studies who have shared their experiences with him; clients from the CTRG that he has had the privilege to work with over the years; and, especially, Steve Regel for his warmth and friendship, and whose vision it was for us to write this book.

Endorsements

'Through my work with Hostage UK and Hostage US, I know all too well the challenges that hostages and their families face. As the authors note, social support and help with the practical challenges of everyday life can make the biggest difference of all to both families coping with the kidnapping of a loved one and hostages rebuilding their lives after release. This is an important book and is essential reading for all professionals helping those impacted by traumatic events.'

Rachel Briggs OBE
Director, Hostage UK and Executive Director, Hostage US

'... just excellent, with everything you wanted to know about trauma in accessible language, we recommended it highly for our peer support officers, counsellors and others providing welfare services.'

Head of Mental Health Services
Police Services Northern Ireland (PSNI)

'This book is a great introduction to post-trauma support and is also, for us, the perfect complement to the peer support Debriefing training provided by Stephen Regel to ICRC staff over the past decade.'

Fabrice Althaus, MD
Head of Staff Health Centre of Expertise,
International Committee of the Red Cross (ICRC)

This book has helped us to enhance the quality of support we offer our clients. It has given us an insight into the challenges faced by those who have experienced traumatic bereavement and as a result we are better equipped to support them through their journey.

Carol North
Homicide Team Leader, Victim Support UK

Contents

Understanding psychological trauma

1

Common responses to traumatic events

➲ Key Points

- The range of reactions following exposure to a traumatic event is wide-ranging, and trauma affects different people in different ways.
- Common responses to trauma include having upsetting thoughts and images, attempting to avoid reminders, feelings of emotional numbness, being on edge and jumpy, and experiencing strong feelings of shame, guilt, anger, and rage.
- When reactions become so distressing and prolonged that everyday life is affected, a person may be diagnosed as suffering from post-traumatic stress disorder (PTSD).
- Some people remain distressed for months and even years after an event, some people return to usual functioning relatively soon, and some may experience a delayed reaction to the event months or years later.
- Exposure to trauma may have a variety of other cognitive, emotional, behavioural, and social consequences, such as relationship breakdown, reliance on alcohol, drugs, or an increase in smoking as a way of coping.
- Traumatic experiences may impair physical health or exacerbate pre-existing physical health problems.

A brief historical introduction

Throughout history, it has been recognized that traumatic events can leave people in a state of confusion, distress, and despair.

> I did within these six days see smoke still remaining of the late fire in the City; and it is strange to think how this very day I cannot sleep at

> night without great terrors of fire, and this very night could not sleep until almost two in the morning through thoughts of fire.

So wrote Samuel Pepys in his diary entry for the 18 February 1667, 6 months after the Great Fire of London in 1666. Pepys's account is one of the earliest documented descriptions of a major disaster and its aftermath. His accounts of the fire and the impact it had on him provide a detailed and fascinating account of the psychological effects of the fire.

Physicians (the disciplines of psychiatry and psychology were still in their infancy) first began to see cases in the nineteenth century of individuals exposed to industrial accidents. The industrial revolution saw the increasing mechanization of industry along with the increase of mechanized travel (e.g. the invention of the railway), which indirectly led to an early study of the impact of trauma. Herbert Page, surgeon to the London and North West Railway in 1883, used the term *nervous shock* and described the effects of traumatic events on individuals following a rail accident thus:

> We know of no clinical picture more distressing than that of a strong and healthy man reduced by apparently inadequate causes to a state in which all control of the emotions is well-nigh gone; who cannot sleep because he has before his mind an ever-present sense of the accident; who starts at the least noise; who lies in bed almost afraid to move; whose heart palpitates whenever he is spoken to; and who cannot hear or say a word about his present condition and his future prospects without bursting into tears.

The author Charles Dickens was a passenger on a train when it crashed in Staplehurst in Kent in 1865. At the scene, he witnessed many distressing sights and helped the injured and the dying. Later when safe in London, he described feeling 'quite shattered and broken up'. Some days later, clearly overwhelmed by his experience, he complained of feeling 'faint and sick' sensations in his head. In a letter to his daughter some years later, he wrote: 'I am not quite right within, but believe it to be an effect of the railway shaking. I am curiously weak—weak as if I were recovering from a long illness . . .' (Ackroyd 2002). He also experienced difficulties in the years following his experience of the crash and developed a phobia of rail travel. Dickens died on the fifth anniversary of the disaster.

The influence of war

Our contemporary understanding of the effects of trauma has been mostly a product of studying the effects of war and conflict on individuals (Abdul-Hamid and Hacker -Hughes, 2014). Perhaps the earliest account of war neurosis was by the Greek historian Herodotus, who described the psychogenic (a person presenting with physical symptoms that are psychological in origin) blindness suffered by the Athenian warrior Epizelus at the battle of Marathon in 490 BC:

Epizelus, the son of Cuphagorus, an Athenian soldier, was fighting bravely when he suddenly lost the sight of both eyes, though nothing had touched him anywhere—neither sword, spear, nor missile. From that moment he continued blinded as long as he lived. I am told that in speaking about what happened to him he used to say that he fancied he was opposed by a man of great stature in heavy armour, whose beard overshadowed his shield, but the phantom passed him by and killed the man at his side.

The British version of the Allied Victory medal depicts the winged figure of Victory on the front of the medal and on the back; it read 'The Great War for Civilisation 1914–1919'. To qualify, an individual had to have entered a theatre of war (an area of active fighting), not just served overseas. Approximately 5.7 million of these Victory Medals were issued.

In the First World War (WWI), terms such as *shell shock* and *war neurosis* were introduced to explain the presentations of soldiers affected by their combat experience. R.G. Rows, a medical physician, wrote of his experiences in the *British Medical Journal* in 1916. He was treating cases of shell shock at the Red Cross Military Hospital, Maghull, Liverpool, and described the following reactions amongst the men he saw:

> In some cases the physical expression of a special emotion, such as fear or terror, persists for a long time without much change. This condition is usually associated with an emotional state produced by the constant intrusion of the memory of some past incident ... they know they are irritable, that they are unable to interest themselves or to give a maintained attention to a given subject ... all this is very real to them and leads to a condition of anxiety which is increased by their not being able to understand their condition; they worry because they fear how far this sort of thing may go.

A seminal paper entitled 'The Repression of War Experience' was published in the *Lancet* in 1918, by Captain W. H. R. Rivers, a physician who began practising as a psychiatrist. Rivers also first worked at Maghull and was subsequently transferred to Craiglockhart Military Hospital near Edinburgh, Scotland, where he began treating patients with what was often referred to as *war neurosis*, his most famous patient being the poet Siegfried Sassoon. River's approach to war neurosis and shell shock was seen as pioneering.

As we know all too well, there have been a number of significant military conflicts since both World Wars. The Vietnam War led to research with veterans suffering from the adverse psychological impact of combat experience. This led to the formal entry in 1980 of post-traumatic stress disorder (PTSD) into the *Diagnostic and Statistical Manual of Mental Disorders, 3rd Edition* (DSM111). The introduction of this diagnostic category stated that war trauma alone was a sufficient condition for long-term disorder. In the

UK in the mid-1990s, there was an increase in public and government interest in the health and well-being of ex-service personnel. This was in part brought about by the D-Day 50-year commemorations and the focus on a generation coming to the end of their lives. There was also the increasing recognition of the psychological impact of trauma following the Falklands conflict. Since then, military psychiatry has developed considerably and has been the focus of a considerable body of research, much of it focused on those service personnel recently deployed in Iraq and Afghanistan. This was partly driven by the large class action brought by a number of Falkland's veterans who claimed the UK's Ministry of Defence had failed to address the issue of PTSD.

So, as we can see, the effects of trauma have long been noted throughout history. But it is only within the last few decades that psychological trauma has become one of the most heavily researched and well-understood topics in psychiatry and clinical psychology (Brewin, 2007). Whilst our understanding of psychological trauma grew from military settings, it was soon realized that civilians caught up in disasters and other tragic circumstances develop the same reactions.

Common reactions to traumatic events

In this book, we will use the word *trauma* to refer to events that are psychologically overwhelming for individuals, families, or communities. These include disasters (technological or natural), war, acts of terrorism, transportation accidents, road-traffic collisions, acts of interpersonal violence, torture, and other events, which are specifically addressed in this book.

Most people are affected in some way when they are exposed to a traumatic event, but their reactions do not last long and are not too distressing. Within days or weeks, most people feel as if they are back to how they were and getting on with their lives. But, for some people, reactions can be more distressing and longer lasting. As we will see in Chapter 3 (Assessment and formulation), there are a number of reasons for this. Some people may be less resilient at that time, perhaps owing to other stressors already in their lives, and so the impact of a traumatic event affects them more significantly. For people who are affected, there is a common core of reactions, and these we will now have a look at.

Much of the time, our lives seem safe and predictable. Serious road-traffic collisions, plane crashes, train accidents, natural disasters, criminal assaults, and other sorts of traumatic events seem to happen to other people, not us. We may read about them in the papers or watch them on TV, but we do not expect to experience them directly ourselves.

But for those of us who have gone through trauma, we know that any of us, at any time, can be the victims of sudden and unexpected tragedies or losses.

Sadly, things can and sometimes do happen to us or to people we are close to, and not just to other people in other places. If they do, we are likely to experience a range of unfamiliar feelings and reactions associated with the shock of the event and may have some difficulty in collecting our thoughts and handling our feelings about what has happened.

There are no 'right' or 'wrong' ways to react, and different people exposed to the same trauma may respond in quite different ways. Everyone's experience will be unique and personal; therefore, the process of psychological adjustment and recovery will differ from person to person.

While most people involved in a traumatic incident will be shaken by what has happened, some adjust to their experiences with little or no apparent distress and emerge emotionally unscathed. This would be considered a quite common response. Sometimes people may in fact feel satisfied by the way that they have acted when faced by the traumatic event (e.g. if they have been able to help others who have been involved).

Other people, however, are shocked and stunned by the traumatic event and have difficulty believing what has happened to them. In the days following the incident, some people feel confused, distressed, and fearful or experience other emotions or reactions, which can in themselves, be unpleasant and worrying. Even though such reactions can seem strange, it is important to understand (and explain) that they are also entirely normal and understandable responses to severe stress and shock. In most cases, the reactions are short-lived and pass after a few days or weeks.

Below are some common feelings, emotions, and behaviours sometimes experienced or displayed by survivors (and sometimes by witnesses, relatives, and emergency workers) in the hours, days, and some weeks following an extremely stressful or traumatic event. These can include any of the following.

Psychological reactions

◆ **Anxiety**—feelings of fearfulness, nervousness, or sometimes panic, especially when faced by reminders of the event; concerns about losing control or not coping; and worry that the situation may recur.

◆ **Hypervigilance**—constantly scanning the environment for cues of danger or seeing threat in things that would have appeared innocent before the trauma. This could mean being overly protective of children or loved ones (e.g. worrying if they are slightly late arriving home or haven't phoned at exactly the time they said they would).

◆ **Sleep disturbance**—difficulty in getting off to sleep, restless sleep, and vivid dreams or nightmares. At first, these may be about the incident itself or the experience, but they can change to be less specific, where the content can just be unsettling or generally disturbing.

◆ **Intrusive memories**—intrusive thoughts/images of the traumatic inci-dent, which can appear to 'come out of the blue', without any triggers or reminders. Other thoughts, images, or feelings may be prompted by media triggers (e.g. something on TV, newspapers, sounds, a song or piece of music, and smells).

◆ **Guilt**—feelings of regret, about not having acted or coped as well as one would have wished, about letting one's self or others down, or about being in some way responsible. Other feelings of guilt may be present because the person survived, whilst a friend or loved one died—again, this is a common phenomenon known as 'survivor guilt'. Often when we feel guilt we want to make things right again somehow.

◆ **Shame or embarrassment**—feelings related to how we think of our-selves, often related to a sense that we were not good enough in some way. When we feel shame, we want to go into hiding.

◆ **Sadness**—feelings of low mood and tearfulness.

◆ **Irritability and anger**—at what happened and the injustice of the event, questioning Why me? at those felt to be responsible for the trauma, and wanting somebody to accept responsibility or blame. Irritability can often be directed at loved ones, close family, friends, or colleagues.

◆ **Emotional numbness or blunting**—feeling detached from others or being unable to experience emotions such love or happiness.

◆ **Withdrawal**—tending to retreat into one's self and avoid social and fam-ily contact.

◆ **Disappointment**—thinking that people (including family) do not really understand how you are feeling.

◆ **Mental avoidance**—avoiding thoughts associated with the trauma. People try to push distressing thoughts out of their head, often unsuc-cessfully, and in the longer term, this can cause further problems because it interferes with the person processing and making sense of their experience.

◆ **Behavioural avoidance**—avoiding thoughts, feelings, and activities that are reminders of the trauma. These can be often subtle at first, such as avoiding noisy or crowded environments, taking a different route to work, and so on. There is also the potential for these avoidances and fears to spread or 'generalize' to other situations; in other words, to experience similar sensations when in situations that have a semblance or resonance to the original trauma. This may mean that someone who feels anxious and avoids driving after a car accident may start to feel anxious and avoid travelling by other forms of transport (e.g. by bus or train) or develop a fear of flying. Charles Dickens, two years after his accident, in 1867, described having 'sudden, vague rushes of terror, even when riding in a hansom cab, which are perfectly unreasonable but quite insurmountable ...'

◆ **An increased startle response**—becoming 'jumpy' or easily startled by sudden noises or movements (e.g. a door slamming shut or the phone or doorbell ringing).

Physical reactions

There may also be physical health problems, including tiredness, headaches, chest pains, gastrointestinal disorders, cardiovascular disorders, renal disorders, respiratory diseases, and infectious diseases, as well as impairments in the immune system. The person may also have certain bodily sensations, with or without the psychological reactions described previously. Many of these symptoms are signs of anxiety, tension, or stress. For example:

◆ Shakiness and trembling

◆ Tension and muscular aches (especially in the head and neck)

◆ Insomnia, tiredness, and fatigue

◆ Poor concentration and forgetfulness

◆ Palpitations, shallow rapid breathing, and dizziness

◆ Gastrointestinal symptoms such as nausea, vomiting, and diarrhoea

◆ Disturbance of menstrual cycle or loss of interest in sex

The course of these common reactions generally takes one of three psychological trajectories.

First, for the majority of people, as mentioned previously, if the traumatic event has not affected them through personal loss or injury or they have not witnessed this in others, they generally tend to regain their sense of equilibrium. This usually occurs within a few weeks. They find that many of their reactions are reducing in intensity, frequency, and duration. These individuals tend to take an 'upwards' trajectory.

Second, others find that their reactions take a fluctuating course and their trajectory is a pattern of 'peaks and troughs', and they find that at times, their reactions are worse or more persistent. This prompts them to become more avoidant of situations, people, or places, which serve as reminders, and this may indeed improve things for a while. However, despite their best efforts, it is not possible to avoid all reminders, so they find it increasingly difficult to predict or control their environment.

Third, for some exposed to traumatic events, the common reactions described continue to worsen, leading to marked avoidance of a variety of situations, which in turn affects their mood, work, relationships, and social functioning. Persons in this group end up on a 'downward' trajectory. These individuals eventually experience moderate to severe PTSD.

Of course, it is too simplistic to say that the event by itself will determine these three trajectories. We now know that pre-trauma factors or 'risk factors', such as a lack of social support, previous trauma, and previous mental health problems will influence the individual's ability to manage the impact of the event. In addition, events that occur in the weeks or months after exposure to trauma also have a significant potential to influence these trajectories. Such events can be described as post-trauma 'complicating factors', and they can present as a diverse range, which could include the scale and nature of the event; ongoing litigation; the impact of injury; the role and involvement of external agencies (e.g. law enforcement agencies, the criminal justice system, and the media); relationship problems, an unsympathetic attitude from an employer; and, of course, the context (social, political, or historical) in which the trauma occurs and the recovery environment.

Therefore, it can be seen that the psychological trajectory or journey that most individuals take is determined by a complex interplay of pre-trauma, event-specific, and post-trauma complicating factors. Inevitably, these will be further complicated if the individual experiences a traumatic loss or losses after the event: this topic will be dealt with in more detail in Chapter 4 (Traumatic Bereavement).

Impact on relationships

As we will see in Chapter 10 (Post-traumatic Growth), in some cases, a shared sense of adversity or loss can bring people closer together, help create new bonds, or strengthen relationships. But, although family and friends are usually understanding and supportive, the experience of trauma can sometimes place strain on relationships.

Trauma may also affect social relationships because of increased levels of irritability, withdrawal, and decreased enjoyment from shared activities, leading to marital and interfamilial discord and sometimes even domestic violence. The person may feel that too little or the wrong sort of help and support is offered or that others do not appreciate what they have been through and expect too much of them. Sometimes, such as in Laura's case, which follows, there may be thoughts of suicide.

🔖 Laura's story

Laura is an experienced mental health nurse who was present when a female patient walked into the day unit she was working in, poured a can of petrol over herself, and then set fire to herself. The patient ran into a toilet and locked herself in. Laura tried for several minutes to save the woman who was on fire, and, despite many attempts, she failed to reach her and prevent her from burning to death. At first, Laura felt that she had coped well with a very traumatic experience and that her experience and training would assist in that coping. However, in the weeks that followed, she found she was experiencing a range of reactions that were becoming more intense and increasing in frequency, intensity, and duration. Her irritability was increasing, especially towards her partner. She was having difficulty concentrating and sleeping, having anxiety and panic attacks, and she felt as though 'she was losing it'. This was most characterized by her extreme reaction one day. 'I was in my bedroom trashing the place and feeling as though I wanted to hurt myself. . . .' Reflecting on her experiences she recalled, '. . . the day after the incident I was offered counselling. I thought, "Why would I need counselling?" Why didn't anyone think to explain how we might feel and what we needed to look out for . . . the last six months have been absolutely awful . . . I never thought I would feel suicidal or want to abandon my partner of 10 years.'

Sometimes, when relationships become strained, there is a tendency for people to rely on alcohol or drugs as a means of coping. In 1987, a passenger cruise ship, the Herald of Free Enterprise, left harbour in Zeebrugge en route to Dover. But, a few minutes out of harbour, water started pouring in through the bow doors, which had not been properly secured. Passengers and crew, oblivious to the danger, were ordering food in the restaurants and settling in to their journey. Without warning, the ship began to lurch and, in less than a minute, it had capsized: 193 people died that day in one of the most horrific maritime disasters of the twentieth century.

A group of psychologists contacted survivors 3 years later and asked them to take part in a survey (Joseph et al. 1992). It was found that amongst survivors:

- 73% reported increased alcohol consumption.
- 44% reported increased cigarette consumption.
- 40% reported increased use of sleeping tablets.
- 28% reported increased use of anti-depressants.
- 21% reported increased use of tranquillizers.

As was noted by Rows (1916), with soldiers from the First World War, the phrase '. . . this is very real to them and leads to a condition of anxiety which is increased by their not being able to understand their condition . . .' has a resonance with many individuals we have seen, who have been exposed to traumatic events. They often do not know what is happening to them or what is common or normal for them in their particular circumstances, something evidenced in Laura's story.

It is again important to emphasize that there are no right or wrong ways to react after a traumatic experience or bereavement. Everyone's reactions will be individual and not everybody will experience all of the feelings described herein, nor experience them to the same degree.

While most people will have at least short-lived feelings of shakiness, jumpiness, anxiety, or anger, some will have either none or milder reactions, dependent on the factors mentioned, including their proximity to the event. However, in the immediate aftermath and following days, if the person has intense or unpleasant physical reactions, sleep disturbance, intrusive memories, feelings of fear or guilt, or other reactions, it cannot be overemphasized that these are entirely common and normal reactions to abnormal events, and, in most cases, are not long lasting.

What is post-traumatic stress disorder?

Whilst it has been noticed that there was a common core to how people react, for some, those whose reactions become more intense, frequent, and upsetting and begin to interfere with everyday life, this can often be the manifestation of what is now known as PTSD (American Psychiatric Association, 2013).

◆ *PTSD* is the term used by mental health professionals to describe reactions that cause clinically significant distress or impairment in social, occupational, or other important areas of functioning in people who have experienced a traumatic event.

◆ A *traumatic event* is defined, in this case, as an event that involves actual or threatened death or serious injury or a threat to the physical health of self or others (e.g. a family member or friend), and, in which, the person felt frightened, horrified, and helpless. This can also include learning about traumatic events that have occurred to close family members or close friends.

◆ In emergency service workers and first responders, PTSD can develop, for example, where there is repeated or extreme exposure to events, such as body handling or repeated exposure to distressing images during the course of their work.

PTSD consists of four clusters of symptoms:

◆ First, when people experience traumatic events, they may have distressing recollections including images, thoughts, and distressing dreams. Many people describe 'flashbacks'. It must be noted here that real 'flashbacks' are often accompanied by a sensory modality, such as touch, taste, or smell, and the individuals feel that they are actually re-experiencing the event as if it were happening again: (e.g. they *feel* as though they are back in the burning car or *can actually smell* the body odour of their assailant). In addition, they may lose a conscious awareness of their surroundings for a few moments or minutes, as illustrated by the following quote from a woman who survived a rail crash: *'I suddenly experience a whooshing sound and feel as if I'm back in the carriage'.*

♦ Second, there are problems with avoidance. When there are reminders, the person may experience distress and feel shaken up. As a result, people often try to avoid reminders, such as thoughts, feelings, or conversations associated with the trauma, or activities, places, or people that bring back memories.

♦ Third, there are negative cognitions and disturbances in mood. Persons may experience changes in beliefs about themselves, others, and the world, leading them to have feelings that others cannot be trusted or the world is a dangerous place. Changes in belief systems about self and the world can lead to feelings of anger, guilt, and shame. People may also shut down mentally and emotionally and have trouble remembering what happened. They may feel cut off from others and have difficulty in having loving feelings.

♦ Fourth, there are problems of arousal. There may also be difficulties falling or staying asleep, episodes of reckless or self-harming behaviour, irritability, or outbursts of anger, hyperalertness, an exaggerated startle response, and difficulty concentrating.

When these problems last for more than a month, a diagnosis of PTSD can be made.

Who is most at risk?

Reactions will vary from person to person, for a number of reasons, including:

♦ Differences in personality.

♦ Ways of expressing emotion.

♦ Styles and methods of coping.

♦ Previous experiences of adversity or trauma.

♦ The extent to which there are existing stresses and strains in other areas of the person's life.

♦ The exact nature of the traumatic event and the individual's or families' experience will also make a difference.

♦ Whether the incident was violent, extraordinary, and unexpected.

♦ Witnessing death and serious injuries.

♦ If the individual was seriously injured, this can also affect subsequent reactions, by numbing or delaying the psychological impact.

No one knows in advance how anyone may react to a particular stressful event. All the same, what happens after extreme stress is to some extent dependent on what was happening in the person's life before the event, what they did during the event, how they dealt with the demands of the situation, and some immediate or early reactions they may have had to their experience.

For instance, if life before the event had been troubled through difficulties within the family, feeling alone, unexpected changes or upheavals, loss or bereavements, or poor health, reactions may be more marked than had circumstances been more favourable. Factors affecting risk and vulnerability, as well as factors that affect the individual's recovery, will be covered in more detail in later chapters. PTSD cannot be diagnosed until at least 1 month has passed since the trauma. This is to recognize that, in the early days, usually the first 6–12 weeks, it is common for people to experience these reactions, and it is only when they become persistent that mental health professionals need to consider formal therapeutic interventions seriously.

Related conditions

The diagnosis for PTSD was developed by the American Psychiatric Association and the World Health Organization (WHO), and the description presented in the chapter is the one most commonly used in the Western world. However, it should be noted that the WHO (1992) also included within its current edition of the International Classification of Diseases a number of related conditions:

1. Acute stress disorder—a condition that develops in an individual following exposure to a traumatic event. Often, reactions may appear, usually within minutes or hours of the event, and often they subside. They are expected to last no longer than 2–3 days at the most. There may be an initial state of 'daze', during which disorientation, panic, and anxiety are commonly present; however, some studies have shown that if this occurs and is sustained over a period of more than a week or so within the first month, it may be a predictor of later PTSD.

2. Adjustment disorder—this refers to states of subjective and emotional disturbance that arise in the period of adaptation to a significant life change or to the consequences of a stressful event, affecting the person's social network through, for example, bereavement. Although it is assumed that the condition would not have arisen without the stressor, what differentiates this category from PTSD is the acknowledgement of the role of individual differences. Symptoms are thought to include depressed mood, anxiety, worry, feeling unable to cope or plan ahead or continue in the present situation, and some degree of disability in the performance of daily routine.

3. Personality changes—these can occur after catastrophic life experiences (e.g. torture, being held hostage, or concentration camp experiences).

Conclusion

It is common to experience a wide range of reactions following exposure to traumatic events, to a greater or lesser extent depending on the event itself, together with the pre- and post-trauma factors described herein. In many cases, symptoms will improve over time. However, some persons exposed to trauma will go onto develop more disabling presentations, which we call PTSD. Commonly, there is fear and avoidance of cues that remind the sufferer of the original trauma. There will be periods of high levels of physiological arousal presenting as panic attacks or other physical symptoms of anxiety.

Negative emotional states are common. As well as guilt and shame, there may be intense feelings of rage and anger. Such negative emotional states are distressing and can lead to destructive behaviours, such as substance abuse, in an attempt to dull or block them. Many people experience symptoms and reactions against the persisting background of a sense of 'numbness' and emotional blunting, detachment from other people, unresponsiveness, and avoidance of activities and situations reminiscent of the trauma.

Rarely, there may be dramatic, acute bursts of fear, panic, or aggression, triggered by stimuli arousing a sudden recollection and/or re-enactment of the trauma (or of the original reaction to it), an enhanced startle reaction, and insomnia. Anxiety and depression are commonly associated with the above-mentioned symptoms and signs, and suicidal ideation may be present. Excessive use of alcohol or drugs may also be a complicating factor.

The effects of trauma can be very long lasting. Studies have shown survivors of disaster and other extreme events, such as sexual assault, remain affected many years later.

Indeed, PTSD has been shown in World War II veterans, those of other conflicts, and survivors of the Holocaust 50 years later. Although problems can exist for many years, people may not be continuously troubled all of that time. A number of people do not present initially, but only months or even years after the event. However, careful assessment often indicates that the person may have been suffering from problems all along, which have varied in intensity, frequency, and duration, but has either not recognized the problem or attributed his or her experiences to other factors.

References

Ackroyd. (2002). *Dickens: public life and private passion*. London: BBC Books.

Abdul-Hamid, W. K., and Hughes, J. H. (2014). Nothing New under the Sun: Post-Traumatic Stress Disorders in the Ancient World. *Early science and medicine* 19(6), 549–557.

American Psychiatric Association (1980). Diagnostic and statistical manual of mental disorders, 3rd ed. Washington, DC: American Psychiatric Association.

American Psychiatric Association (2013). Diagnostic and statistical manual of mental disorders, 5th ed. Washington, DC: American Psychiatric Association.

Brewin, C. (2007). *Post-traumatic stress disorder: malady or myth*. New Haven: Yale University Press.

Joseph, S., Yule, W., Williams, R., and Hodgkinson, P. (1993). Increased substance use in survivors of the Herald of Free Enterprise disaster, *British Journal of Medical Psychology* 66, 185–191.

Page, H. W. (1883). *Injuries of the spinal cord*. London: Churchill.

Pepys, S. (2003). *The diaries of Samuel Pepys: a selection*. (New ed.) London: Penguin.

Rows, R. G. (1916). Mental conditions following strain and shell shock. *British Medical Journal* 1, 441–443.

WHO. (1992). *The ICD 10: classification of mental and behavioural disorders: clinical descriptions and diagnostic guidelines international classification of diseases*. Geneva: World Health Organization.

2

Concepts and theories
of post-traumatic stress

➲ Key Points

- Theories provide us with ways of understanding peoples' reactions to traumatic experiences.
- Biological, behavioural, psychodynamic, social-cognitive, and integrative psychosocial theories are reviewed.
- Psychologists, psychiatrists, and counsellors use theory to formulate and plan therapy.

Introduction

In this chapter, we discuss the theories of trauma. Much theoretical work has been carried out in the field of psychological trauma, since the concept of post-traumatic stress disorder (PTSD) was first introduced. A variety of theories of psychological trauma has been put forward.

We will examine the main theoretical perspectives that have been presented for understanding trauma. First, we review the biological perspective. Second, we look at the concept of emotional processing as proposed by Rachman. Third, we discuss the psychodynamically informed information-processing approach of Horowitz. Fourth, we examine social-cognitive ideas surrounding 'shattered assumptions' put forward by Janoff-Bulman. Fifth, we describe the dual representation theory proposed by Brewin and colleagues, and the cognitive model of PTSD as developed by Ehlers and Clark. Finally, we discuss the integrative psychosocial approach of Joseph, Williams, and Yule.

The aim is to provide the reader with a sketch of the different theoretical perspectives. Although it is beyond the scope of the present book to provide a comprehensive examination of each perspective, readers will be equipped with knowledge that will be useful to them in making sense of their own or other peoples' reactions, and in talking things through with health professionals.

Biological perspective

A good starting point is the recognition that post-traumatic stress reactions, such as being in a state of constant alertness, having an excessive startle response and focused concentration, are characteristic of a special 'survival mode' of functioning. There are three types of responses: flight, fight, or freeze.

Parts of the brain are thought to be activated when individuals are exposed to traumatic situations to allow the flight or fight mechanisms to be activated, and that means that some people are not able to 'switch off'. In traumatic situations, a variety of biological processes are activated. Pupils of the eyes dilate; the heart beats faster; the rate of breathing increases; and blood flow increases and is redirected to the muscles for quick movement. These are the reactions of the sympathetic nervous system, which prepares people for action—flight or fight. A key feature of PTSD, however, is that these reactions continue in the absence of any real danger, given that the original threat has passed.

These reactions are controlled by the brain's limbic system or, more specifically, the amygdala (the brain's 'gatekeeper' for incoming emotional information). In normal circumstances, information is passed from the amygdala to the frontal cortex, such that people can process what is happening and create memories. In threatening situations, however, it is thought the amygdala passes information directly to the hypothalamus (the cortical memory centre), releasing chemicals that stimulate the fight-or-flight response but that circumvent the normal route to learning and the storage of memories. The amygdala also receives numerous connections from the hippocampus. Since the *hippocampus* is involved in storing and retrieving explicit memories, its connections to the amygdala may be the origin of strong emotions triggered by particular memories.

As such, persons who survive traumatic events are likely to remain in a high state of alert, experiencing vivid, intrusive, but unprocessed images and thoughts, until the body's fear system is deactivated and they are able to engage again in normal processing. There is still a lot of research going on into how the brain works, and although much is still not known, two parts seem really important in coding memories during trauma. The amygdala has very fast connections with the senses, like sight, sound, and smell. It lays down a memory that is sensory and emotional.

Many people who have a dog will know that sometimes it may bark without any apparent reason. The amygdala acts a bit like a guard dog, so if something looks, smells, or sounds a bit like the trauma (e.g. you hear a sound such as a siren) then the amygdala 'barks', sending warning messages to the rest of your brain, bringing images to mind and making you jumpy and fearful. However, while fast, and necessary for survival, it can be like a dog that barks for no apparent reason.

Then there is another part of the brain called the hippocampus, which stores the meaning and context of what's happening, a kind of story that includes what happened, when, and what it all meant. This is slower to operate but is cleverer. This is a bit like the dog's owner. When the whole system is working properly, the two parts (guard dog and its owner) communicate well. So, for example, when a siren is heard, the guard dog may be about to bark, but the owner reassures the dog that the sound is not dangerous. The owner lets the dog know that 'It's alright, this time the siren is different, the trauma is not going to happen again'. Many traumatized persons are unable to regulate this fear signal, and the arousal continues.

This of course is very different to experiencing fear and other symptoms where threat and danger is ever present, such as in situations where there is ongoing civil conflict, persistent threat as in domestic violence, and other similar situations. In situations where there is continuous traumatic stress, then states of constant alertness, having an excessive startle response and so on, make sense, as the person is prepared to react in survival mode.

In essence, the biological perspective is that PTSD is caused by the biological mechanisms that are activated during trauma, and which are adaptive during trauma, but somehow fail to switch off once the danger is past. So the person remains in survival mode.

From a biological perspective, it could be seen that individuals who display marked symptoms of post-traumatic stress have been biologically primed to respond to danger where none exists. The emotion of fear is a normal and characteristic emotional response to threat and danger, and this in turn is influenced by our memory of what represents threatening situations or what they have meant in specific instances in experience and in our past.

But when it is not possible to fight nor flee, the only alternative is to submit. The third type of response is freeze. This may serve a protective purpose and, occasionally, when individuals are faced with significant threat a phenomenon known as dissociation, which may occur around the time of the traumatic event and can lead to a variety of sensations, such as thinking that time has slowed down and things are moving in slow motion or losing awareness of one's surroundings.

In freeze, the reactions of the parasympathetic nervous system are to decrease heart rate and respiration, lower blood pressure, and so on, such that in extreme situations, individuals go into a state of stupor called tonic immobility. In this state, there is conscious recognition of what is happening, and events can be observed with sensation or emotion. It is thought that this is an instinctive survival mechanism that evolved to protect us in times of danger because tonic immobility may fool predators into not taking further action, or, in a more contemporary scenario, it may convince a gunman to walk on.

Such reactions are likely adaptive, as they enable people to respond to dangerous situations, thus increasing the chance of survival. From an evolutionary perspective, post-traumatic reactions might be adaptive in many situations and might therefore be considered a normal and adaptive reaction. A similar evolutionary significance might be attached to the protective function of dissociation when stress exceeds coping resources' capacity. However, the persistence of reactions and their interference with everyday social functioning are problematic.

The work of Pierre Janet

These ideas discussed herein thus far, can be traced back to Pierre Janet (1859–1947), who originally embarked upon his professional career as a professor of philosophy but later became interested in the phenomena of hypnosis and rose to great prominence in international psychiatry during the turn of the twentieth century. Despite dying in virtual obscurity, and many of his ideas being swept away by Freud's teachings, which became the principal psychological theory of much of the twentieth century, Janet is now seen as one of the seminal thinkers and contributors to our understanding of the impact of trauma on individuals. Janet thought that people exposed to traumatic events suffered from a loss of capacity to store and utilize conscious information.

Janet (1911) suggested that intense emotional reactions cause memories of particular events to be dissociated from consciousness and to be stored as visceral sensations (panic and anxiety) or visual images (nightmares and flashbacks). These intense emotions interfere with the integration of the experience into existing memory schemas. Janet considered dissociation, in the context of trauma, to result from a state of physiological hyperarousal, which results in memory disturbance. Dissociation can be described as a range of processes that involve 'the destruction of the usually integrated feelings of consciousness, memory, identity and perception of the environment' (examples of dissociation will be given in Chapter 3). The information conveyed by the traumatic event is not available to ordinary conscious representation and so cannot be processed. Instead, it persists as a fixed idea that is split off from consciousness and experienced in nightmares.

Janet described how keeping these memories at a distance used a great deal of mental energy, leading to continuing deterioration.

Janet believed that the initial emotional reaction to the traumatic event (which he referred to as 'vehement emotion') dictated the intensity of post-traumatic reactions. He believed that when people get very upset they stop being able to make sense of an experience and can no longer work out what action to take to escape. Modern studies have supported Janet's belief that post-traumatic reactions originate in 'vehement emotions' that are biologically encoded. Contemporary research also supports the idea that the initial level of physical arousal predicts the severity of the response. For example, in a study that followed survivors of an oilrig disaster in the North Sea of Scotland, it was found that the severity of dissociative symptoms predicted longer-term distress.

Rachman's emotional processing theory

Turning now to the behavioural perspective, one idea that we find very useful is 'emotional processing'. Psychologist Stanley Rachman introduced this idea in 1980, before the term *PTSD* was formally introduced.

What Rachman did was to observe that many different emotional and behavioural reactions experienced by people, such as grief, nightmares, and obsessions, could all be understood as manifestations of a failure to process emotionally an upsetting experience. The concept of emotional processing, therefore, provides a powerful theoretical perspective with which to understand a diversity of seemingly unrelated phenomena. Thus, when the concept of PTSD was introduced, with its hallmark symptoms of re-experiencing, avoidance, and hyperarousal, Rachman's theory allowed us to conceptualize PTSD as indicative of incomplete emotional processing.

Rachman's theory suggested that we have a need to absorb emotional reactions. So, following a trauma, there may be a lot of emotional confusion and distress, but, over time, most people are able to absorb their emotional reactions. However, not everyone does so, and that's when we see post-traumatic stress reactions, such as upsetting dreams, nightmares, and so on. Rachman (1980) writes, "Broadly, successful processing can be gauged from the person's ability to talk about, see, listen to or be reminded of the emotional events without experiencing distress or disruptions." He proposed various factors, which give rise to difficulties in emotional processing. Events that are sudden, intense, dangerous, uncontrollable, and unpredictable are harder to absorb emotionally. People with a more anxious personality, who are in a state of fatigue, who have other stressors in their lives, and who have problems expressing themselves will have difficulties emotionally processing or making sense of extremely stressful events.

The emotional processing theory of Rachman can help us understand how people are able to return to pretrauma states. In summary, his approach provided three important perspectives. First, a conceptual framework that helps us to understand a range of previously disparate phenomena; second, that people have some form of intrinsically motivated drive towards processing powerful new emotional information; and third, that processing itself could be promoted or impeded by various events, personality, activity, and emotional states.

Horowitz's information-processing theory

Moving to thinking derived from the psychodynamic perspective, Mardi Horowitz provides what we think is another useful way of understanding trauma. Horowitz's approach is based on the idea that people have mental models, or beliefs, about the world and themselves, which they use to interpret their experiences. He also proposes that there is an inherent drive to make our mental models coherent with current information (what he called the 'completion principle'). In this respect, Horowitz's theory is similar to that of Rachman in proposing that people have some innate need to 'work through' or process emotional experience.

Horowitz (1976) says that a traumatic event presents information that is incompatible with existing beliefs. This incongruity gives rise to a stress response requiring reappraisal and revision of the schema. As traumatic events generally require massive changes in worldview, complete integration and cognitive processing take some time to occur. During this time, active memory tends to repeat its representations of the traumatic event, causing emotional distress; this manifests itself as the intrusive re-experiencing of the event. Re-experiencing symptoms mean that the person is in the process of working through, but this is distressing, and, therefore, prolonged re-experiencing can be too much for the person so he or she moves into an avoidant phase to prevent emotional exhaustion.

Thus, there is a process of inhibition and facilitation, which acts as a feedback system modulating the flow of information. The symptoms observed during stress responses, which Horowitz categorizes as involving denials and intrusion, occurring because of opposite actions of a control system that regulates the incoming information to tolerable doses. If inhibitory control is not strong enough, intrusive symptoms, such as nightmares and flashbacks, emerge. When inhibitory efforts are too strong in relation to active memory, symptoms indicative of the avoidance phase occur (see Figure 2.1).

Typically, avoidance and intrusion symptoms fluctuate in a way particular to the individual without causing flooding or exhaustion that would prevent adaptation. The person oscillates between the states of avoidance and intrusion until a relative equilibrium is reached when the person is said to have worked through the experience. The emotional numbing symptoms are thus viewed as a defence mechanism against intrusion. Horowitz suggests that there are phases of intrusion and avoidance as the person gradually doses himself or herself with information.

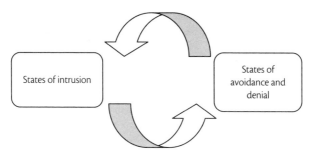

Figure 2.1 Denials and intrusion occur as a result of opposite actions of a control system

So, intrusive and avoidant states characteristic of post-traumatic reactions are to be expected in the aftermath of a traumatic event, as the person emotionally processes his or her experiences. But, not everyone successfully works through his or her experience, and for some the process can get stuck. While intrusive memories are a universal phenomenon indicative of a normal process of working through, over time, if emotional processing is unsatisfactory, then persistent memories represent the failure of emotional processing. The longer the time elapsed since the trauma, the more likely intrusive thoughts will predict poor outcome.

In summary, the information-processing approach of Horowitz draws our attention to the central role that memory plays in the development of post-traumatic stress reactions. The completion tendency maintains the trauma-related information in what Horowitz refers to as active memory, causing it to intrude into consciousness in the form of flashbacks, nightmares, and unwanted thoughts, as the individual endeavours to merge the new information with pre-existing models of the self and the world. In essence, the completion tendency serves as the driver for processing to take place. Such an approach is, therefore, compatible with Rachman's concept of emotional processing: Both emphasize that post-traumatic stress reactions are signs of incomplete processing and both point towards an intrinsic need to absorb and integrate trauma-related information regarding the event.

Janoff-Bulman's social-cognitive approach

Trauma has been referred to as the 'atom smasher' of personality. Janoff-Bulman's social-cognitive approach suggests that there are common psychological experiences shared by victims who have experienced a wide range of traumatic situations. She proposed that post-traumatic stress following victimization is largely due to the disruption of three core assumptions about, the world, self, and others: (1) the world as benevolent, (2) the world as meaningful, and (3) the self as worthy. Coping with victimization involves the person coming to terms with these shattered assumptions and re-establishing a conceptual system that will allow them to function effectively. For example, most of us are trusting of people we meet, and that is why con artists are able to trick people into parting with their life savings for scam investments. Those who have been tricked in this way may find their assumptions about benevolence sorely challenged.

If we are on holiday and relaxing on a beach, we don't expect, as happened in 2015 in Tunisia, a gunman to appear and start shooting. Such an event challenges our expectations and assumptions about the world as meaningful. Our assumptions are shaken up—resulting in the symptoms of PTSD as we try to make sense of what has happened.

Or imagine, a parent is late for work, and because of this, is irritable that morning with his or her daughter, who goes off to school in tears. On the way, the daughter is hit by a car as she is crossing the road. The parent blames him or herself, and his or her sense of self as worthy is shattered.

Drawing on Horowitz's theory, Janoff-Bulman's (1992) approach accommodates the notion of the completion tendency, and that people are intrinsically motivated to make sense of and find meaning in their experiences. Janoff-Bulman proposes that there is extensive mental rumination and processing as persons attempt to make sense of their experience and re-establish their worldview. She distinguishes between automatic processes and intentional efforts to restructure what she described as our assumptive world.

Dual representation theory

Emotional processing involves both 'verbally accessible memories' (VAMs) and 'situationally accessible memories' (SAMs). VAMs we can deliberately retrieve from our store of autobiographical experiences. SAMs contain information that cannot be deliberately accessed by the individual and are not available for editing.

Therefore, SAMs, as the name suggests, are accessed only when aspects of the original traumatic situation cue their activation, e.g. a sight, sound, or smell. These are represented within a completely personal context and they contain sensory information (e.g. taste and smell) and other information concerning personal meanings about the traumatic event. For example, someone who was injured in a terrorist bomb attack in a city centre is watching television one evening when he sees a news report containing a similar violent episode to the one he experienced. In that moment, his SAMs are accessed, and he experiences the same smell of burning flesh that he did in the original attack.

VAMs are characterized by their ability to be deliberately retrieved and edited by a traumatized individual. It is argued that VAM representations contain the sensory, response, and meaning information about the traumatic event. Talking through one's experiences with a therapist allows VAMs to be activated, and thus edited and elaborated.

This theory proposes that VAM and SAM representations are encoded in parallel at the time of the trauma, and between them, they account for the range of PTSD symptoms. Brewin and colleagues (1996) proposed that individuals need to consciously integrate the verbally accessible information in VAM with their pre-existing beliefs and models of the world, and thereby restore a sense of safety and control through making appropriate adjustments to expectations about their self and the world.

Cognitive model of PTSD

Ehlers and Clark (2000) developed a cognitive model of PTSD. They propose that persistent PTSD only develops if an individual processes the trauma in a way that causes them to experience a sense of ongoing current threat. This threat might result from reliving symptoms (e.g. flashbacks), the impact the trauma has had on his or her perception of the world (e.g. the world is not a safe place), negative appraisals of the self during the trauma (e.g. I could have prevented this), or negative appraisals of the self post trauma (e.g. I'm a useless person because I am not coping). The emotion that most readily corresponds with the notion of threat in PTSD is fear; however, the model proposed by Ehlers and Clark allows attention to be paid to other emotions and the role these might play in the development of ongoing current threat. They suggest that current ongoing threat can be seen as external, such as seeing the world as a more dangerous place (fear), or internal, such as seeing oneself as a less capable or acceptable human being. Such appraisals can generate strong emotions: one that is particularly relevant is the emotion of shame. It has been proposed that shame can act as an internal current threat by attacking the individual's psychological integrity, leaving them feeling inferior, socially unattractive, and powerless, thereby maintaining his or her PTSD symptoms.

Psychosocial approach

In Joseph, William, and Yule's (1997) psychosocial framework, it is proposed that traumatic events present people with information that, as perceived at the time, gives rise to extreme emotional arousal. Representations of these event stimuli are held in memory because of their personal salience and the difficulty they present for immediate emotional processing. These event cognitions will idiosyncratically reflect the individual's personality, environment, and social context.

Event cognitions can then form the subject of further cognitive activity called appraisals. Appraisal cognitions are distinguished from traumatic cognitions in being thoughts about the information depicted and its further meanings.

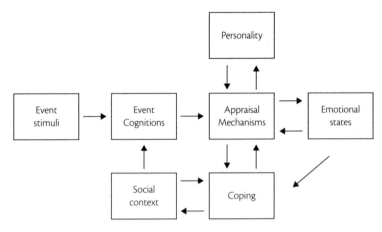

Figure 2.2 The psychosocial framework of post-traumatic stress reactions

How one appraises an event is influenced by personality, emotional state, and coping. Any stimulus is capable of being perceived in a variety of ways: what is dangerous to an inhabitant of Manhattan may not seem so to someone who has lived on the Ganges and vice versa.

Appraisal processes lead to various emotional states (e.g. fear, panic, grief, guilt, and shame). The occurrence of these event appraisals and emotional states will all engender attempts at coping, which may either be active problem-solving strategies or avoidant thoughts and behaviours.

In this model, which is schematically represented in Figure 2.2, individual variation is attributable to a complex interaction between components that constitute variables that may contribute to outcomes at different points in time. What is helpful about this framework is that it provides a way for therapists to help clients develop an understanding of why their difficulties have arisen and to formulate a plan for change, as we shall illustrate next in the story of John.

Using theory to plan for change

Theory helps clinicians think about the problems that people experience following trauma, as well as how to help. To illustrate, John was in a road traffic collision in which his fiancée died. Although it was not John's fault, he blames himself for what had happened. This reflects John's personality, which is more pessimistic than optimistic. As a result, he feels ashamed and guilty. As a result of these feelings, John tries to avoid thinking about what happened and avoids other people who he feels will judge him. Over time, he becomes socially isolated, in part because of his own avoidance, and in part, because other people don't know how to react and withdraw from John to minimize their own discomfort (see Figure 2.3). Over time, this becomes a

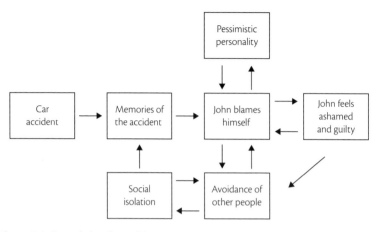

Figure 2.3 Formulating the problem

self-perpetuating cycle of appraisals, emotional states, and coping, in which John becomes mired down in shame and guilt, socially withdrawn, and increasingly depressed, with thoughts of taking his own life.

John is referred to the psychologist who helps him understand his cycle of appraisals, emotional states, and coping, and how, over time, they have fed into each other and led to a downward spiral into depression. Together they discussed ways in which John could change in order to put the cycle into reverse. A programme was developed involving cognitive therapy to challenge John's pessimistic thinking, in order to build his personal resources to deal with his negative appraisals, alongside a behavioural intervention to teach John new skills in coping and seeking support (see Figure 2.4). Gradually, as John practices his new skills, he is able to increase his social support and challenge his negative thinking.

The psychosocial framework shows how different personal and social factors influence each other in such a way as to lead to distressing thoughts and unhelpful behaviours. Think of how all the components of the psychosocial framework can conspire to produce a downward and vicious cycle for people in which they become more and more self-defeating, self-blaming, withdrawn, isolated, and so on, leading to the maintenance of post-traumatic stress symptoms and the emergence of new emotional problems such as shame, guilt, and anger.

Recent work by Joseph, Murphy, and Regel has taken the psychosocial framework a step further and used it to describe how therapists can help clients not only halt any such downward and destructive cycle but reverse it to create an upward and constructive cycle in which all the components conspire together to create positive changes—commonly referred to as post-traumatic growth (see Chapter 10).

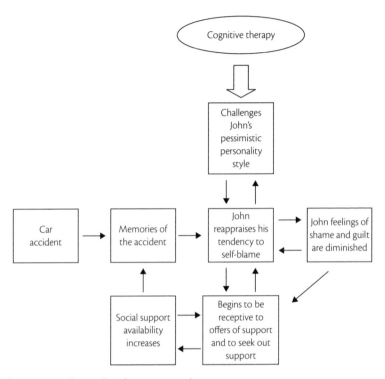

Figure 2.4 Understanding the treatment plan

We will return to the topic of formulation in Chapter 3, when we will discuss in more detail the factors that are important in determining outcomes and how this influences choices for treatment.

Conclusions

Theories offer us a pair of spectacles through which to look at psychological trauma. In this chapter, we have discussed different theories, from the biological underpinnings of trauma reactions, through cognitive explanations, to the interaction of personality, coping behaviours, and social support processes. Each theory offers us something different. Theory is useful, and therapists will use it to help them and their clients make sense of their experiences and plan appropriate and adaptive interventions.

References

Brewin, C. R., Dalgleish, T., and Joseph, S. (1996). A dual representation theory of post-traumatic stress disorder. *Psychological Review 23*, 339–376.

Ehlers, A. and Clark, D. M. (2000). A cognitive model of posttraumatic stress disorder. *Behaviour Research and Therapy 38*(4), 319–345.

Horowitz, M. (1976). *Stress response syndromes*. New York: Jason Aronson.

Janet, P. (1983) [1911]. *L'etat mental des hysteriques*. 2nd ed. Marseille: Lafitte.

Janoff-Bulman, R. (1992). *Shattered assumptions—towards a new psychology of trauma*. New York: Free Press.

Joseph, S., Murphy, D., and Regel, S. (2012). An affective-cognitive processing model of post-traumatic growth. *Clinical Psychology and Psychotherapy 19*, 316–325.

Joseph, S., Williams, R., and Yule, W. (1997). *Understanding post-traumatic stress: psychosocial perspectives on PTSD and treatment*. Chichester: Wiley.

Rachman, S. (1980). Emotional processing. *Behaviour Research and Therapy 18*(1), 51–60.

3

Assessment and formulation

⮕ Key Points

- The majority of people will experience at least one traumatic event in their lifetime.
- Most people are affected in some way by trauma but are quickly able to return to their normal state. However, some people develop severe and long-lasting problems.
- Post-traumatic stress disorder (PTSD) can occur at any age, including childhood.
- Men tend to experience more traumatic events than women do, but, often, women experience events of higher impact.
- Women are more likely than men are to develop PTSD in response to traumatic events.
- Social support is a significant protective factor following exposure to traumatic events.

The prevalence of trauma reactions and PTSD in the community

How common is PTSD? Estimates suggest that around 1 in 10 women and 1 in 20 men will develop PTSD at some point in their lives. There may be a number of reasons for this difference. For example, men and women may experience different types of traumatic events.

Some traumatic events are associated with particularly high rates of PTSD. For example, rape has been associated with the highest PTSD rates in a number of research studies, as have childhood neglect, physical and sexual abuse, physical attack, and being threatened, kidnapped or held hostage. The types of traumatic event that people experience will also vary with age.

Following the most traumatic events, it is thought that around 40% of the people involved are likely to develop PTSD. For other events, the percentage will be lower, and for most events, it is estimated that only around 8% of people will develop PTSD. As such, most people who are exposed to a traumatic event do not go on to develop PTSD or other problems, such as anxiety, depression, and other psychiatric conditions. Individuals, families, and communities can often cope effectively following exposure to traumatic events by using their own resources.

The most important resource is social support from community, friends, families, workplace colleagues, and so on. When we have strong social support, we are most able to buffer what life throws at us.

We also know that persons who lack resources such as social support are more likely to develop problems. Other findings from the research on PTSD in the community indicate that the people most at risk of developing post-traumatic reactions include:

♦ Those exposed to/or who have witnessed extreme traumatic events, such as physical and sexual abuse, natural or human-made disasters, road-traffic collisions, serious crime, or military action.

♦ Those considered special 'at-risk' populations, such as emergency service workers (e.g. police and ambulance personnel) are often more likely to have an increased risk of exposure and could, therefore, be at higher risk of developing post-traumatic reactions. Therefore, occupational health and welfare departments in the emergency services must pay close attention to the welfare of such groups (see Chapter 8, Early Intervention Strategies: Mental Health Promotion).

♦ Many refugees and asylum seekers have also experienced a range of traumatic events, such as rape, torture, acts of organized violence, and other physical abuse, including witnessing such events, and are, therefore, likely to suffer psychologically because of this exposure. However, the topic of refugees is dealt with in Chapter 7 (Cultural Responses to Trauma) in further detail because culture can be an important mediator in terms of the manifestation and presentation of post-traumatic reactions.

But, even in such high-risk populations, not all develop PTSD or other problems. Why do post-traumatic stress reactions develop in some but not in others, and what maintains the symptoms, such as re-experiencing the event, high levels of anxiety, and avoidance, which are often significant problems for many, for long periods?

Why do some people develop PTSD and some do not?

It is an intriguing question for many researchers and practitioners as to why some people will go on to develop psychological problems and PTSD following exposure to traumatic events and others do not. This is where an understanding of risk factors is helpful. Often, the stressful or traumatic event itself is rarely enough to produce problems in many of those exposed. A case in point here would be emergency service workers and others exposed to, what for many would be, extreme, harrowing, traumatic stressors on a daily or weekly basis, yet, often, they do not go on to develop problems. We will return to some of these issues later.

In general, there are three main categories of risk factors that often dictate the individual's psychological trajectory following exposure to traumatic events (as mentioned previously in Chapter 1, Common Reactions to Traumatic Events). These are:

◆ Pre-trauma factors

◆ Peri-traumatic factors (i.e. specific phenomenon that occur around the time of the event)

◆ Post-traumatic factors—these can also be described as complicating factors, as there are a number of issues that can arise following exposure to a traumatic event that serve to exacerbate the individual's or family's psychological journey in the wake of a traumatic event.

Whilst a number of risk factors have been identified, the specific risk factors are often not as clear-cut as it would seem. In a number of cases, many do not have any of the pre-trauma risk factors previously identified, and yet they go on to develop a range of post-traumatic symptoms and PTSD following exposure to a traumatic event. These are often specifically related to the peri-traumatic risk factors and are often concerned with the individual's idiosyncratic meaning of the experience.

Pre-trauma risk factors

Whilst a number of pre-trauma risk factors have been identified, the most significant would be:

◆ **Previous stressors**—these could also be described as 'life events', such as bereavement, ongoing relationship difficulties, ill health, work-related stress, and financial difficulties.

◆ **Previous psychological problems**—these could range from previous episodes of anxiety and/or depression, family history psychiatric problems, or history of trauma or childhood abuse.

Peri-traumatic risk factors

Prei-traumatic factors occur around the time of the traumatic event.

♦ **The person experiences a sense of loss of control** over themselves or events around the time of the trauma.

♦ **Subjective life threat**—this refers to the common experience that many people have when exposed to a severe or significant traumatic event, which is that they are going to die. The event would involve exposure to death, serious injury to the individual, or a near miss.

♦ **Guilt**—there are usually two forms of guilt: one is related to what is often described as 'acts of commission or omission', in other words, the individual will perceive, often erroneously, that they did or did not do something that then led to the event occurring or to someone coming to some harm. The other form of guilt is known as 'survivor guilt', whereby the individual feels guilt at surviving the experience, when a loved one, colleague, friend, or others did not.

♦ **Peri-traumatic dissociation**—this phenomenon can occur when individuals are exposed to high levels of threat. Dissociation is often characterized by individuals describing phenomena, such as 'time having stood still', and 'it seemed like it went on forever, but it must have been a few seconds'.

Perhaps the best way of describing the experience of peri-traumatic dissociation is to give two examples. The following is from the explorer David Livingstone, who described his reactions when engaged in shooting a lion, which attacked him whilst he was loading his rifle. He goes on to report the lion bringing him to the ground, growling, and shaking him. He described the shock of the experience as producing a stupor similar to that which seems to be felt by a mouse after the first grip of the cat. 'It caused a sort of dreaminess in which there was no sense of pain or feeling of terror, although I was quite conscious of all that was happening....'

A woman, who had been involved in a train crash where there had been a number of fatalities and injuries, also described a similar phenomenon as follows.

> I was aware of someone on top of me as I couldn't move but I felt no pain and was euphoric and quite elated, even though I had a head wound. I wasn't aware of anybody else on the train only when I looked over my shoulder and saw this pile of bodies....

Another form of peri-traumatic dissociation can be found in Eric Lomax's book, *The Railway Man*, an autobiographical account of his experiences as a Japanese prisoner of war in Burma. In his book Lomax describes his disorientation in terms of his altered sense of time following his interrogation at the hands of his captors. He describes emerging from an episode of interrogation, which he thought had lasted all night, into what be believed to be the dawn sunlight but then realized it was setting sun.

Post-traumatic risk factors

As indicated previously, post-traumatic risk factors (which can also be described as complicating factors) can influence the outcome of an individual's psychological recovery. These can include a whole range of elements that are often interrelated.

- **Social support**—studies have often shown that levels of social support relatively soon after a traumatic event can often predict the way symptoms develop over the forthcoming months. Therefore, social support, especially the quality and accessibility of it, can be a major protective factor following exposure to traumatic events. The type of social support can be informational, practical, and emotional, and it may vary according to the individual's needs over time. It is important to match the provision to the needs of the affected individuals, families, or communities.

- **Substance misuse**—the use of alcohol and drugs in the immediate aftermath of a traumatic event as a way to deal with the impact can also affect the recovery process.

- **Acute stress reactions or acute stress disorder (ASD)**—as indicated in earlier chapters, an acute response following exposure to a traumatic event has been shown to be predictive of problems in the longer term.

- **There may also be financial considerations**, often linked to physical injury, requiring frequent hospital visits, surgery, and a loss or change of employment.

- **A perceived lack of justice** in the wake of a traumatic event, which can be caused by the way the individual is dealt with by their employer, a social agency, or even by a range of historical, social, and political events, such as those experienced by many following the Troubles in Northern Ireland, as one example. Whilst the political situation has changed dramatically in Northern Ireland, over the past decade, for many, there remain feelings of guilt, shame, anger, and rage at the events that took place.

- **The scale and the role of the media** can often affect an individual's recovery, as there will often be frequent reminders through the written and visual media, through documentaries or newspaper and magazine articles. Often people are asked to give interviews about their experiences, and these have the potential to harm in perhaps subtle and less obvious ways than first imagined. For example, their stories and experiences may be misrepresented because of factual inaccuracies. They may also be exposed to other aspects of their experience, which may serve to re-traumatize them when they are at their most vulnerable.

♦ **Accumulative traumatic events** can also be seen as another complicating factor, as the individual's exposure to repeated events, which may take their toll over time, finally culminate in an experience that is ultimately too much for the person to deal with. People often say things like, it was the 'straw that broke the camel's back', meaning that they were managing despite all that had happened, and then something else happened. Often, that event they would have normally coped with, but it just added to the weight of everything else, thus affecting the capacity to cope.

Often there may be no obvious risk factors present, but the individual develops problems because of various factors that occur after the event, as in the following example of Jill's story.

📃 Jill's story

Jill was a passenger in a train crash. She was a 38-year-old happily married professional and was 39-weeks pregnant. She had no pre-trauma vulnerabilities. During the crash, Jill wedged herself on her back between a seat and table, fearing that if the violently shaking train window shattered, she would fall through it and die horribly. On arrival at the hospital, A&E staff did not find the baby's heartbeat, although an experienced midwife later did. She then spent 24 hours strapped to a monitor listening for a change in the baby's heartbeat, which might indicate placental damage. Two weeks later, her baby was born normally and healthy. But, she spent those 2 weeks fearing her baby was dying; she took her concerns to midwives who checked for the unborn baby's health but did not pick up on Jill's growing anxiety. Once her baby was born, she started having nightmares (including 'out of body' experiences) about her baby being dead or them both being trapped in wreckage (which had not happened in the crash).

These nightmares spilled over into her waking life; she saw danger everywhere. She suffered debilitating feelings of sorrow when terrible events happened to other people and, gradually, she could not cope with the world. She became very withdrawn, was utterly exhausted, and was signed-off sick from work for a few weeks. She returned to work, which in hindsight she knows was far too early and ended up taking a second period of sick leave.

She had a strong belief that, as she was not physically injured, she should just 'get over it' and 'get back on the horse'. So, for about 18 months after the crash, she tried to continue travelling on trains but was effectively re-traumatized on each occasion. She saw an admission that she had been affected by the crash as evidence she was 'not a strong person' and had a 'weak character'.

She now refers to these views as a prejudice (but one she felt is deeply entrenched in a very 'British attitude') that contributed to her withdrawal. Eighteen months after the crash, she began attending weekly counselling, which initially focused on helping her accept that she had been injured, albeit psychologically, and on overcoming her feelings of shame (we will return to Jill's story in Chapter 9, Treatment for Post-Traumatic Stress).

The assessment

For many trauma sufferers, the assessment process is a difficult and painful process. They will have to discuss events, experiences, and memories that they have been trying to avoid, often for many years. However, it is the responsibility of clinicians to treat them with great sensitivity and address their concerns about the process. The therapist needs to acknowledge that the assessment may cause the individual significant discomfort, and should reassure them that it is an 'information-gathering' process. The assessment will enable the therapist to find out as much about the trauma and the impact it is having on the individual's life, in order to be able to help the individual try to make sense of and come to terms with their experience. Once that information has been gathered (and this may take more than one appointment), appropriate therapy should be discussed. Patients should be given plenty of opportunity to discuss what is on offer in the way of therapy and whether or not they feel it is the right approach for them at that time in their lives.

At this point, it must be said that there are different therapeutic approaches to helping trauma sufferers and that therapists with different orientations will approach the assessment process differently (Wilson and Keane, 1997). The assessment approach described in this chapter is cognitive behavioural therapy (CBT), which is recommended in the National Institute of Clinical Excellence in Health (NICE, 2005) Guidelines for The Management PTSD in Adults and Children in Primary and Secondary Care. However, it may not suit everyone, and other approaches will be discussed. The therapist using this model will also use questionnaires to aid the assessment process, and these will be discussed later. The assessment is an extremely important initial contact, as it allows the therapist to develop a rapport with the trauma sufferer, gain a thorough understanding of the person, the problem, and his or her journey since the trauma, and to determine whether this approach will work for the person.

Assessment of post-traumatic stress

Research has highlighted the need for thorough and comprehensive assessment. Many individuals are referred to specialist psychological therapy or trauma services with the minimum of information. Therefore, the referral letters may contain very little information about the nature and impact of the traumatic experience. Patients may have previously seen a number of mental health professionals (psychiatrists, community psychiatric nurses, or social workers, counsellors or psychotherapists) and described their experience many times over. This may or may not have been of benefit and, indeed, some of the problems may have resolved and others may have worsened. When interviewed about their problems, patients may often not display any degree of distress or emotion. However, this can be misleading because they may have recounted their experiences many times, and hence, it can seem like telling a story. It may be done with a level of detachment and disassociation, which may belie the distressing and debilitating nature of their traumatic experience. Often, this may occur simply because patients may have never been asked the appropriate questions in the context of (a) the diagnostic criteria for PTSD or (b) within the framework of the theoretical models underpinning our understanding of the development of post-traumatic reactions and (c) any considerations of complicating factors or co-morbidity (this refers to the presence of other conditions such as depression). Therefore, a multifaceted approach to assessment is advocated, which needs to include the following questions:

- Why this person?
- Why this problem?
- Why now?

The assessment also allows the therapist to make a formulation about the person's problem and then provide a rationale as to why he or she feels the approach may work. Additionally, the therapist would then explain what the therapy would entail, as well as the anticipated or expected outcomes.

Whilst CBT is collaborative in nature, it is often challenging and demanding. The importance of establishing a good rapport and relationship cannot be understated.

Pre-trauma history

- Establish the individual's previous levels of functioning.
- Determine the person's baseline of functioning.
- Examine the common themes of the individuals life struggles or conflicts.

Immediate pre-trauma psychosocial context

It is extremely important to assess the trauma victim's psychosocial context at the time of the trauma: for example, what was the individual's age and level of development? What life events was the individual dealing with at the time? What was the level of development of the person's family system?

The event and immediate coping responses

◆ Was it single or multiple trauma?

◆ Were the traumas clearly delineated incidents?

or

◆ Was the trauma a culmination of a number of experiences?

◆ Was trauma human-induced or an act of nature?

◆ Did it occur to only one individual, the family, or a group?

Active/passive role

◆ Was the person a helpless victim or did he or she perceive his or her actions as such?

◆ Was he or she active in any way to alter the situation?

◆ Were there any options for acting differently?

◆ How does the patient perceive the meaning and outcome of his or her actions?

Meaning of the trauma

This is extremely important because traumatic experiences can have specific idiosyncratic meanings for the individual. This would be dependent on a variety of factors, such as thoughts and imagery at the time the trauma occurred.

Post-trauma psychosocial context

Areas of consideration should be the presence of ongoing stressors (e.g. the individual is acting as the main carer for an elderly, confused relative or is experiencing relationship problems or going through other significant life events) and the responses of the family, the community, and social agencies.

◆ Family responses—often the family or close friends of trauma sufferers may not understand what is happening to the loved one or friend. Because no one wishes to cause those close to them further emotional distress, family members may unwittingly encourage avoidance of situations, places, or people. Moreover, family members may appear to respond unsympathetically by becoming irritable with the person because they do not understand what is happening to him or her and perceive his or her behaviour as unreasonable.

◆ Responses from social agencies—various social agencies may be involved in the aftermath in providing help, but as with family and friends, it is possible that agencies can themselves unwittingly cause further distress and confusion, particularly where there is a lack of communication between agencies and with the survivors and their families.

Other areas to consider are:

◆ Was the patient treated with respect?

◆ Was the patient satisfied with treatment?

◆ Were there elements of secondary victimization? In other words, did the patient experience other difficulties in the wake of the event, such as problems being re-housed, receiving criminal injuries compensation, or have difficulties with receiving insurance entitlements?

An example here is of a young couple who had put their savings into renovating a small terraced cottage in a former mining village. The cottage was on the main road near a sharp bend. One night whilst watching TV, a car containing four teenagers and being driven at speed ploughed into the living room of the house after the driver lost control of the vehicle. A young man in the passenger seat died at the scene. The couple not only witnessed this, but it was some considerable time before they were rescued from the house. Later, after repairs were completed, cracks started to appear in the inner walls, and the house was deemed unsafe. The insurance company argued that as their house was an old property, they were ineligible to receive compensation for their loss, and this led to a protracted and expensive legal dispute.

Assessment of attribution and meaning

◆ What are the person's new views of self and the world?

◆ Are there new personal outlooks in place?

◆ What does the trauma mean in terms of the individual's plans for the rest of his or her life?

◆ Is the person focused on the unfairness of the past or on the possibilities of the future?

Assessing strengths and resources

◆ When does the person feel better (even when it is only the exception and not the rule)?

◆ What thoughts, feelings, and behaviours does he or she have at those times?

- Which coping strategies tried have been (even partially) successful?

- What other difficult situations has the person overcome in the past?

- What resources were called upon at that time?

- Who does the person see as providing him or her with support in times of difficulty or crisis?

Asking about social support

One of the important things the therapist should try to do is to understand what social support the person has in his or her life. (Joseph, Andrews, Williams and Yule 1992). Some things to consider asking patients would be:

- Do they have people who are able to offer them emotional support?

- What about practical support?

- Have the people they thought they could rely on rallied round to help or do they feel let down and isolated?

- Were people supportive at the beginning, but their offers of support seem to lessen over time?

- Are they able to reach out to others and ask for support when they need it?

By asking such questions, the therapist is able to initiate a conversation about support, as well as how patients use it. Not everyone makes the best use of the support available. What the therapist should do is discuss ways in which patients can make better use of their support.

Evaluate the degree to which the person believes:

- A response exists that will alleviate their suffering.

- It is within their power to perform the response.

It would also be appropriate to ask about alcohol consumption and a typical drinking week, assessing alcohol intake in units. For alcohol and drugs, change in patterns and amounts following the event need to be considered. Similarly, questions should be asked about prescribed or non-prescribed drugs, and information should be sought regarding current or past medication. Assessments are best conducted using face to face interviews, however information can be supplemented by self report questionnaires prior to treatment commencing. There are a number of useful questionnaires appropriate for post traumatic stress and associated conditions e.g. depression, which are also useful to audit clinical changes (Fischer and Corcoran, 2007). These will be described in more detail in Chapter 9, Treatment for Post Traumatic Stress.

At the end of the assessment

An appropriate course of action needs to be considered, depending on the experience and expertise of the therapist. This would be to:

◆ Deal relatively soon with high levels of anxiety or arousal or other distressing symptoms.

◆ Offer advice, guidance, and education (see Chapter 9), depending on the length of time between the assessment and the trauma (e.g. if within the first 6–12 weeks, then offer follow-up appointments at regular intervals to assess progress). A reasonable time frame would be at about 1 month, 3 months, and then 6 months.

◆ If the person is beginning to have difficulty coping and needs more intensive therapeutic intervention, this should be initiated at this point and more targeted, trauma-focused CBT or other therapy, as appropriate, should be considered.

References

Fischer, J., and Corcoran, K. (2007). *Measures for clinical practice and research: a sourcebook.* 4th ed. Oxford: Oxford University Press.

Joseph, S., Andrews, B., Williams, R., and Yule, W. (1992). Crisis support and psychiatric symptomatology in adult survivors of the Jupiter cruise ship disaster. *British Journal of Clinical Psychology*, 31(1), 63–73.

Lomax, E. (1995). *The railway man.* London: Jonathan Cape.

National Institute of Clinical Care Excellence (NICE). (2005). *Guidelines for the management of PTSD in adults and children in primary and secondary care.* London: Gaskell.

Wilson, J. P., and Keane, T. M. (1997). *Assessing psychological trauma and PTSD.* New York: Guilford Press.

Responding to trauma in different contexts and settings

4

Traumatic bereavement

> ## ➲ Key Points
>
> - Traumatic bereavement occurs after a sudden, violent, and unexpected loss. It carries the potential for longer-term psychological problems for the bereaved.
> - Formal counselling and therapy in the first few weeks or months often is not indicated for the majority of those bereaved in this way.
> - Early social support, providing information and guidance about common reactions to traumatic bereavement and the course of those reactions in a structured manner, can be helpful to the bereaved.
> - Providing affected persons with practical strategies to manage daily and future challenges is an important part of early social support. Such support has the potential to protect the bereaved against complex longer-term grief reactions and other adverse psychological complications.
> - Emotional social support from others, whether family, friends, or professionals, who are willing and able to listen empathically to the bereaved person, will be helpful in most cases.
> - Some general guidelines are provided for those who may be called upon to provide support in the early stages of such bereavement.

Introduction

Any bereavement or loss is traumatic. However, *traumatic bereavement* occurs when the loss is sudden, violent, and unexpected, and often, those affected experience a loss of control over events. There is a potential for longer-term problems, depending on the circumstances and nature of the loss. The experience of being involved in a traumatic bereavement, whether it is following death in a road traffic collision, house fire, homicide, manslaughter, act of terrorism, or natural or technological disaster, can happen to anyone, anywhere, and at almost any time, as evidenced by past and recent events involving significant losses of life. Many individuals and families who have experienced such bereavement find that their profound loss and grief are compounded by a variety of factors, which often seem beyond their control. This random element makes the experience terrifying and shocking, particularly because the individuals cannot prepare or indeed protect themselves from the effects of the traumatic event.

📖 Mark's story

Mark and Jason, aged 14 and 18, respectively, lived with their mother following their parents' separation. Nevertheless, the relationship between their parents seemed amicable, and they enjoyed equal contact and good relationships with both parents. One day they arrived home from school to find both parents dead in the kitchen. They learnt later that their father had stabbed their mother and then killed himself. The reasons for the murder/suicide were never clearly established.

Their father had a large extended family that had accepted their mother as one of their own. Inevitably, there was significant shock and horror in the family at the death of the parents, and the prime concern was for the welfare and well-being of Mark and Jason, who were not only bereaved but also witnesses to the scene. Within 2 weeks of their loss, the boys were included in meetings held with the whole family. The meetings were structured along the model of structured social support, as outlined in Figure 4.1. Meetings were held individually with key members of the family, and then with each of the boys. Information was provided, paying close attention to specific examples that the family had described and discussed. It was soon clear that Mark was struggling with recurring imagery, but he was provided with some self-help and other coping strategies. He was carefully monitored, and gradually the imagery diminished over time. Mark's school was also contacted and informed about the nature of the support he was receiving, which staff members clearly found helpful. Jason also received some individual support meetings, but soon left for university. Contact was maintained with the family, including both boys, throughout the inquests and funerals, usually at fortnightly intervals. Contact was maintained with Mark for about 2 years, but with decreased frequency. At the last meeting, he had clearly made significant attempts to come to terms with his loss. He was doing well in his studies, had maintained good relationships with his extended family and friends, and continued to have a close relationship with his brother. Overall, Mark and his family were seen for 18 appointments in total.

Accessing early support following a traumatic bereavement can make a significant difference in the long-term recovery of individuals and families affected by such events (De Leo, Cimitan, and Dyregrov 2013). This chapter summarizes some of the common reactions that occur after such traumatic events, the course of these reactions, complicating factors, and some strategies that may help to manage the impact of the many challenges that arise consequently. Moreover, a section provides guidance for those providing support for individuals and families bereaved in such instances.

The process of grief and mourning

The experience of loss is common to all our lives, and many individuals encounter repeated losses over their lifetime, in many ways. In some cases of traumatic loss, an individual or family may lose several family members in a single event. Grief is expressed in a wide variety of ways and is a natural reaction to a significant loss. The experience of grief fluctuates over time. There is no 'right or wrong' way to grieve, and there is a great variability in how people respond to the death of a loved one. For example, grief may increase or decrease depending on a variety of factors, such as life events, anniversaries, reminders, or events that have a resonance because they are similar to the person's own experience. The grieving process has many phases, and whilst there are many different ways of describing this, one way of viewing the process is to think of it as consisting of stages: numbness, shock, disbelief, and feeling overwhelmed, followed by disorganization, yearning, despair, and hopelessness, and then, in time, straightening up the mess and ultimately reinvesting and re-engaging with life. This description describes a typical sequence; however, everyone is different, and the duration of each stage and the sequence in which it occurs can vary from person to person. It is common for survivors to feel a profound sense of emptiness, a loss of interest in the world around them, and hopelessness about the future. Essentially, *grief* is reacting to the loss, and *mourning* is the active process of reorientation and adjustment over time, the 'reinvesting and re-engaging' with life.

As we saw in Chapter 2, the experience of traumatic bereavement can also shake or shatter the individual's (or family's) 'assumptive world'. Meaning that, as human beings, we hold three basic beliefs or assumptions about the world, others, and ourselves. These are often described as 'silent assumptions', as we are not conscious of holding these beliefs: in general, these are (a) a belief about personal invulnerability, (b) a sense that the world is meaningful and comprehensible, and (c) a positive sense of ourselves and others. The experience of traumatic death can shatter a person's assumptive world or everything that the person holds to be true about his- or herself and the world. This is why in an individual, family, or community, following an experience of traumatic bereavement, there is a profound sense of violation, confusion, and loss of identity and meaning, as if the world has been turned upside down.

Common reactions following a traumatic bereavement

Following the exposure of individuals or families to a sudden traumatic bereavement, it would be very common, and of course completely understandable, for those affected to experience a range of reactions (to a greater or lesser extent). Of course, many factors determine the extent to which these reactions may be present. For example, factors that may affect the course of such reactions could include the age of the deceased, the relationship with the surviving family, the nature of the death, the degree and impact of media involvement, the involvement of other agencies (e.g. the health and justice system of one's own or other countries, depending on where the event occurs).

As with any traumatic event (discussed in Chapter 1), a variety of common reactions follow the experience of traumatic bereavement, but there are also a number of differences. Some of the most common reactions following traumatic bereavement may be:

- Profound feelings of sadness, helplessness, anger, rage, shock, and numbing

- Feelings of guilt or shame, whether over acts of omission or commission (e.g. individuals feeling that their actions or even decisions made before the event may have contributed to the death of a loved one or a friend); often these thoughts and feelings are based on information the bereaved have after the event rather than before, a phenomenon often described as 'hindsight biased' thinking; many describe survivor guilt (described further in the section on 'psychological reactions' in Chapter 1)

- A continued pervasive fear associated with the dread of anticipated violence towards self or others, coupled with a strong sense of vulnerability

- Surviving relatives and loved ones may display compulsive behaviours of self-protection

- Strong feelings of constant hypervigilance (also described in the same section in Chapter 1)

- Constant 'what if?' or 'if only . . . ' thoughts, but these become very unhelpful over time and lead to very unhelpful thinking patterns—as a relative once said to me, 'the "what ifs" are the road to hell, as I soon came to realize, there is only "what is"'

- A compulsive need for a tangible reassurance of a family presence and safety of other family members

- Concerns about the reactions of other family members, especially those of elderly parents or siblings

- Behaviours and emotions directed towards retribution by the perpetrators

- Some may experience reconstructed memories of an event that they have not witnessed

- Difficulty sleeping, waking during the night, and finding it hard to return to sleep

- Impaired concentration and finding it hard to stay focused on tasks at work or at home

- Irritability, which can create friction with others who do not understand this as a traumatic reaction to the bereavement

- Mental and behavioural avoidance of reminders of the event

Families affected by traumatic bereavement can at times feel isolated and stigmatized within their communities. Bereavement and loss will affect members of the same family in different ways, leading to different coping strategies. These can sometimes disrupt or fracture the infrastructure of the family unit and change close and extended family relationships. Significant changes can occur in the structure and dynamics of the family: for example, in the case of a family with four children (a girl aged 17, two boys aged 14 and 10, and a girl aged 5), bereaved by a serious road traffic collision, where the mother and youngest child were killed. The eldest daughter became the oldest woman in the family, and the younger of the boys now became the youngest member of the family instead of being a middle child.

Research indicates that it can take up to 2 years before many individuals can begin to find their sense of equilibrium again, and individuals and families often have many additional challenges to face during that time. The sheer shock of the loss, combined with a number of external complicating factors, will often severely interfere with or inhibit the usual coping mechanisms of even the most resilient individuals.

At the time of writing, many victims and bereaved families in the UK affected by the terrorist shootings in Tunisia are having to contend with a range of stressors brought about through their ongoing involvement with the security services, police, and national and international legal and justice systems. The flow of information can be inconsistent, and affected people have to deal with information that is highly graphic and traumatic, such as coroners' reports. Further, they will have to handle the financial affairs (which in some cases may be complex), inquests, decisions regarding memorials, and other related matters for the deceased. Given the inevitable differences in the wishes and opinions in families, this can also present an added stressor.

Many of those affected may often also find themselves unable to continue to work for a variety of reasons, such as the constant demands described previously. Therefore, a return to work that is graded, gradual, and supported by the employer will help individuals to adjust to new challenges and stressors. Employers need to be made aware of the significant impact of such traumatic losses and be empathic to the period needed before return to the work place (helpful information for employers can be found at the end of the book).

Some who are bereaved may also have to deal with severe economic hardship, and worry over managing financial affairs, with which they are unfamiliar. Preoccupation with the traumatic event can also, naturally (and sometimes seriously), disrupt normal parenting patterns. This in turn can contribute to confusion and distress in surviving children, and, at worst, to truancy and antisocial and criminal behaviour, which can be exacerbated by the child's own experience of the original event (e.g. witnessing the loss of a sibling or parent). In some cases, any pre-existing vulnerabilities among surviving loved ones can be exacerbated by the loss.

In the majority of cases, the sudden death of a family member is not witnessed by the person's loved ones; often, they are notified of the loss by a phone call or a knock on the door. If the death is witnessed or survivors were in close proximity and perhaps under threat themselves, survivors have the potential to develop complex problems such as post-traumatic stress disorder (PTSD), compounded by feelings of guilt, which can become entrenched and intractable if support is not offered in within a few weeks of the loss. Of course, the greater or more significant the event, the greater the person's risk of developing of mental health problems (Dyregrov, Dyregrov, and Kristensen 2014).

What helps in the early stages of a traumatic bereavement?

◆ Studies have found that, in many cases, early interventions and support are effective in reducing long-term psychological complications These studies have shown that family members affected by extreme traumatic events and traumatic bereavement benefit by:

◆ Early help supplying information, guidance, and support

  ◆ Outreach help

  ◆ Information about the event and potential reactions

  ◆ Help over time

◆ An opportunity to meet with others who have experienced similar situations (Dyregrov 2001).

Studies have also demonstrated that crisis interventions delivered through an approach that involves the provision of information, guidance, and structured social support can help individuals and families recognize and manage their reactions and the many challenges they will have to face. Early structured support can also help them manage their expectations of themselves and others following the bereavement.

So what is meant by 'early interventions' or 'structured support'? As mentioned earlier, in the majority of cases, formal counselling or therapy is not indicated, especially in the first few weeks. Often following trauma, there is a powerful need to talk, so, rather than therapy, a form of intervention known as 'structured social support' should be considered. It may be helpful for people in working through their experiences, helping them to process and come to terms with their loss. This can be invaluable for people as they search for meaning in their experience. The importance of social support cannot be emphasized highly enough because this, rather than formal therapeutic or counselling approaches, will be of greatest help to those affected by traumatic bereavement. Further, there is a significant amount of evidence indicating that the provision of social support is a protective factor following exposure to extreme stressors and trauma—conversely, a lack of social support is a strong predictor of long-term problems.

The process of providing 'structured social support'

This section will be useful to those called upon to assist individuals and families affected within weeks of a traumatic bereavement. Assessment of the individual, family, and children (if appropriate), is paramount, and it can be conducted in a number of ways. One method would be to conduct a series of meetings (e.g. with the family as a whole, with individual members, and with children, if necessary and where appropriate) to assess natural resilience and sources of social support. The importance and role of assessment cannot be overemphasized. Assessment and re-evaluation should be cyclical processes (see Figure 4.1) to take account of the changes in family circumstances and other developments brought about by the continuous traumatic stressors and changing dynamics within the family that are a common features of a traumatic bereavement (e.g. constant press attention, legal proceedings, coroners' inquests, and new [and possibly distressing] information coming to light as a result of any investigation or ongoing proceedings, legal or otherwise).

The role of assessment is a crucial step in deciding whether any formal therapy is indicated. In many cases, continuing normal reactions within the context and circumstances of the bereavement would be assessed. If individuals begin to display specific trauma symptoms or show signs of developing serious mental health problems after 6 months, they should be referred for further assessment in the first instance, through their general practitioner. When assessing the impact on children, specialist input should be sourced, and it is often helpful when working with a family, to collaborate with a co-therapist. In addition, consideration

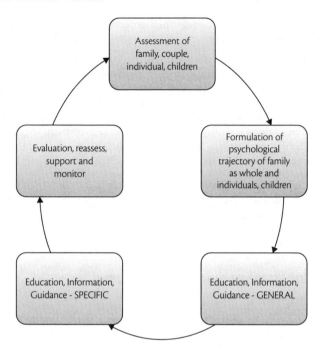

Figure 4.1 Structured social support: the process

and preparation needs to be given to upcoming anniversaries and other important occasions that may affect the family (Stroebe et al. 2008).

One of the key considerations in the early phases is the process of 'normalization'. The rationale for providing information about usual reactions, the course of those reactions, and coping suggestions close to a critical event is that it is often helpful for people to know the landscape they will subsequently inhabit. This can help minimize feelings of alienation and help people understand that others in the same situation will be experiencing similar reactions. Research has shown that misinterpretation or negative appraisal of one's own reactions can contribute to the development of a marked lowering of mood, heightened levels of anxiety, and conditions such as PTSD. Therefore, providing explanations that help contextualize the event and one's own and others' reactions is believed to mitigate against further problems.

Information can be provided within the first few weeks. Typically, during the first few days and weeks, people are overwhelmed by their loss and are less receptive to information. It is important, therefore, when supporting someone within a few weeks of bereavement, to provide information with caution. When providing education, information, and guidance about common reactions, an educational framework that emphasizes contextual factors should include consideration of the following factors:

- Education regarding the impact of a traumatic bereavement, common reactions, and the course of those reactions, within the context of the individual's or families' experience

- Discussion of the emotional and physical reactions, within the context of the individual's and families' experience

- Advice and expectations about managing fear cues, intrusive thoughts, and reminders, using examples from the individual's/family's own experience e.g. 'media triggers' from TV or other media sources. It is also helpful to highlight the strong possibility that subsequent events that have a resonance with the families' own experience, such as hearing about events very similar to their experience, will have the potential to reactivate distressing memories and emotional responses to the original event e.g. if they have been victims of a terror attack, hearing about similar incidents will trigger further feelings of anxiety or fear.

- Advice about dealing with mental and behavioural avoidances—give specific advice concerning 'adaptive versus maladaptive responses'; for example, advise self-monitoring to pick up any gradual but consistent avoidances of triggers and reminders; if these become entrenched, then more serious psychological problems can ensue; advice regarding confronting reminders and fear cues should be exercised with caution, especially in the early stages as individual resilience; access to regular support and regular therapeutic monitoring will play a part in the way an individual processes this aspect of support

- Discuss the predicted time frame of emotional reactions and any influencing factors based on contextual circumstances

- Discuss self-care (e.g. following a routine, structuring the day, and maintaining family rituals)

- Highlight the possibility of changes in outlook and attitude and the impact this can have on coping strategies

- Encourage the use of other support services (e.g. self-help groups and third-sector provision)

- Recommend the use of appropriate reading or self-help literature

- Meeting others with similar experiences (this should also be arranged after careful consideration through organizations experienced in the specific nature of the bereavement, and be monitored carefully and closely)

- The inclusion of other information, advice, and guidance specific to the nature of the bereavement

Meetings should be informally structured because this provides a sense of 'safety' and containment. It may be helpful in some cases to give the individual/family a brief written bullet pointed summary of either (a) each meeting or (b) after a series of meetings because it can be difficult to retain information when under conditions of continuous stress. Our experience indicates that many of the points listed above need to be reinforced on a regular basis.

If therapy or counselling that is more formal is indicated, a trauma-focused CBT (TF-CBT) approach may not suit everyone. It would be important to assess the presenting circumstances and discuss individual needs and preferences. At this stage, other approaches, such as client-centred counselling that offers empathic listening and acceptance may be more helpful, as those approaches will offer the bereaved the opportunity to make sense of their loss and its significance to them.

Some may indeed benefit from TF-CBT at a later stage if it is clear that they are suffering from marked depressive symptoms or in some rare cases PTSD symptoms. Usually, the development of PTSD symptoms, such as frequent intrusive thoughts and images, nightmares, re-experiencing the event, flashbacks, and other symptoms are more likely to occur (a) if individuals have witnessed the death of a loved one, (b) if they are exposed to graphic images and details as a result of reading formal post mortem documents or attending the trial, or (c) begin to develop memories based on information they have been told about the manner of the death. This phenomenon is sometimes known as a 'reconstructed memory', such as in the example of a mother (see Sandra's story) whose two young children were hung by her husband, who then subsequently hung himself. She had regular nightmares for many years, of three shadowy figures hanging on an upstairs landing—she did not witness the scene, and the family lived in a bungalow, but she had constructed a memory of the event from fragments of information that continued to manifest in regular nightmares of that specific content for several years until she had psychological treatment.

📄 Sandra's story

In 1988 Sandra experienced a traumatic bereavement following the murder of her two children aged 1 and 4, by her husband, who also committed suicide following the murders. There was every indication that he had also planned to murder Sandra. Throughout her relationship, she was subjected to serious physical, sexual, and psychological abuse. Her coping mechanism was to engage in regular sporting activities, especially swimming. Sandra worked as a swimming instructor for many years before suffering a back injury after a fall at work in 2003. She is now registered as disabled and needs regular physiotherapy and painkilling injections.

Despite being seen by a number of mental health professionals over the past 26 years, her trauma symptoms continued, particularly marked avoidance of several situations, and recurrent nightmares.

Nevertheless, she remarried and now has a supportive husband and two grown-up children from her present marriage. Since attending therapy, her symptoms have markedly diminished, and she is gradually coming to terms with her traumatic bereavement responses. For example, she is now able to look at photographs of her deceased children, display these at home, and openly discuss the events of the past. She has increased her level of independence and she is far less reliant on her husband for day-to-day functioning. She travelled to town for the first time in 23 years alone and often travels to the trauma centre alone. She also continues to swim as regularly as possible.

Sandra has always acknowledged that had she received support at an early stage following her bereavement, she would have coped more effectively with the challenges she has faced over the years.

Finally, many individuals who have experienced a traumatic bereavement have described instances where the counsellor or therapist has actively avoided any active or in-depth discussion of the circumstances surrounding the trauma or bereavement, because they themselves have found the material difficult or distressing. Many have noted the counsellor's visible emotional discomfort upon hearing the disclosure of difficult material, sometimes becoming openly tearful. This will heighten or add to the affected individuals' or families' distress, causing them to either 'censor' or minimize the impact of the trauma, which inevitably inhibits the narrative and thus their ability to begin making sense of their traumatic loss. Additionally, it leads to a loss of trust and confidence in the counsellor's professional credibility. Therefore, whilst not actively encouraging individuals to describe their experiences if they do not wish to do so, there should be an honest discussion of what degree of disclosure would be comfortable. The practitioner should also have extensive experience in working with traumatic bereavement because this will facilitate the provision of a 'safe' environment and contain the often painful and at times graphic disclosures made in such sensitive encounters.

Conclusions

◆ Following a traumatic bereavement, it is common to experience a range of reactions, which are often normal under the circumstances. Normalizing these reactions can reduce feelings of alienation and assist with processing the traumatic event and losses.

◆ Assessment of individual and family resilience, the presence (or absence) of social support, and past coping styles can often predict the psychological trajectory.

◆ Education and information provided should always take account of specific contextual factors.

◆ Structured social support as described herein, should be provided in an empathic manner, with a practical and pragmatic approach that takes explicit account of people's natural resilience.

◆ Formal therapy or counselling should not be considered in the first instance. Rather, a discreet process of continual assessment and evaluation will highlight any need for formal therapeutic interventions when appropriate.

◆ If formal therapy is indicated, then assessment for evidence-based collaborative approaches such as TF-CBT should be considered. Whilst, TF-CBT will facilitate working through the meaning of loss, and its significance is important, some people may benefit from alternative approaches.

◆ Practitioners experienced in dealing with traumatic bereavement on a regular basis should provide both early interventions through the provision of structured social support and later therapy if indicated.

References

De Leo, D., Cimitan, A., Dyregrov, K. et al., eds. (2013). *Bereavement after traumatic death: helping the survivors.* Gottingen: Hogrefe.

Dyregrov, K., Dyregrov, A., and Kristensen, P. (2014). Traumatic bereavement and terror: the psychosocial impact on parents and siblings 1.5 years after the July 2011 terror killings in Norway. *Journal of Loss and Trauma: International Perspectives on Stress and Coping.* 1–21. doi: 10.1080/15325024.2014.957603

Dyregrov, K. (2001). Early intervention – a family perspective. *Advances in Mind-Body Medicine* 17, 160–196.

Stroebe, M. S., Hansson, R. O., Schut, H., and Stroebe, W. (2008.) *Handbook of bereavement research and practice: advances in theory and intervention.* Washington, DC: American Psychiatric Association.

5

Taken hostage

Some considerations for victims, families, and employers

> ### ⊃ Key Points
>
> ◆ The threat and experience of being taken hostage has increased over the past 2 decades.
>
> ◆ Many individuals and families who have had a loved one taken hostage will experience a range of reactions that although normal in the circumstances, will nevertheless benefit from consistent support.
>
> ◆ Those affected by hostage situations will often experience ongoing traumatic stressors because of the uncertainty, and will benefit from structured social support.
>
> ◆ Employers need to consider the health, well-being, and welfare of their employees' families.
>
> ◆ Hostage situations are long, drawn out, complex, and unpredictable and may have tragic consequences; therefore, hostages' families need consistent information and support from a variety of agencies.
>
> ◆ Support for individuals and families affected by kidnap situations is available through specialist charitable organizations.

Introduction

The last 2 decades have seen the continued and frequent use of kidnapping as a tool used for political and financial motives. Kidnapping in areas such as the Middle East, Somalia, Yemen, Pakistan, Afghanistan, and Nigeria have been reported. Many Western kidnap victims are employees of multinational industries (e.g. journalists, staff and personnel from foreign consulates, and foreign nationals) caught up in any ongoing political crisis or merely in the wrong place at the wrong time. In addition, aid workers who were once deemed 'off limits' are no longer safe from kidnapping, as multiple recent events have demonstrated. Tragically, as the world has witnessed recently, a number of these abductions have ended in the murder of the hostage.

The history of hostage taking is a long one. Only recently, have there been serious attempts to study the effect of hostage situation on individuals and their families. The psychological impact of being held hostage has been well documented, both in the academic literature and through personal accounts, such as those of Terry Waite, who wrote about his experiences in his memoir *Taken on Trust*. Whilst there have been studies on groups of hostages, much of our knowledge is based on what we know about the impact on individuals, often from high-profile cases such as those of Terry Waite, John McCarthy, Brian Keenan, and James Foley.

How such kidnappings affect the families of those who are taken is less well understood because the research is sparse. However, it is likely that close family members are often considerably affected and may develop significant psychological problems in their own right as a result of the uncertainty and fear surrounding what will happen to their loved one.

We will attempt to describe some of the issues that arise for individuals and families. We will also briefly discuss how sensitive and proactive organizational responses can make a difference in helping and supporting kidnap survivors and their families come to terms with their experience and assist them in coping with often life-changing circumstances. Many of the issues discussed in the chapter will also be appropriate and relevant for those who have suffered a traumatic bereavement (see Chapter 4).

The effects on the individual

As with any traumatic event, the impact of being taken hostage will to a great extent depend on a number of factors, including the duration; the nature of any assault on the abducted, whether it be psychological, physical, or sexual; any subjective life threat (i.e. did the individual feel at any point that he or she was going to die); whether the experience was endured alone or as part of a group; the behaviour of the perpetrators; and the whole meaning of the experience for the individual, which will of course determine their psychological trajectory over time. Individual reactions to being taken hostage include many of the following:

- Shock, numbing, and denial
- Fear and anxiety
- Helplessness and hopelessness
- Anger
- Guilt
- Confusion and disorientation

- Impaired concentration, memory, and decision making
- Social withdrawal
- Mental and behavioural avoidance

All these reactions will fluctuate and may occur in phases or be prolonged depending on individual circumstances. Many reactions are similar to those of a traumatic bereavement (as described in Chapter 4).

Family reactions and responses

The first reaction of the families and friends of a kidnapped person is inevitably a mixture of fear, anxiety, and helplessness, which can rapidly degenerate into frustration and anger if the recovery process is slow or seems to be non-existent, and in many cases, the recovery process is often both a slow and torturous one. For organizations that have to deal with this early stage, it requires a great deal of tact, patience, and know-how to deal with the friends and families and avoid making a difficult situation even worse. Much like the hostages themselves, families are forced into a position where they have almost no control over the most important events in their lives at that moment, leading to feelings of anxiety, helplessness, and panic. In many cases, family coping and problem-solving strategies combined with extant family resources, such as communication, support, and flexibility help families to cope in a crisis. As mentioned in previous chapters, there is a significant body of evidence showing that meaningful social support, whatever the source, is a key protective factor following extreme stress and trauma.

What should the responses of organizations and employers be in such situations?

The organization needs to have three key objectives in reference to the families: alleviate their suffering, maintain their trust, and maintain the organization's operational effectiveness (Rudge and Regel, 2014). The consequences for failure can result in families ceasing to cooperate with organizations, seeking their own solution to the problem, engaging in their own media campaigns, or blaming the organization for negative outcomes. Even in the case of a positive outcome, families who feel they have not been treated right by employers can become a long-term public relations problem. In the wake of a kidnapping, families in a state of acute distress find themselves meeting a whole new range of officials: those from the foreign ministry of their country (in the UK this will be the Foreign and Commonwealth Office), the Police, security services, insurers, private security companies, and, of course, their loved one's employers. This can be a bewildering array of individuals, who, despite their best and valid intentions to help, can overwhelm a family that has been suddenly projected into a world of ongoing traumatic stress.

Given the chaotic and traumatic situation in which families find themselves, it is vitally important that the immediate response is one of consistency, reliability, and honesty. As a first step, identifying a consistent individual organizational point of contact is crucial. This, of course, can be one or two individuals who can provide consistent support throughout the whole experience. The UK-based charitable organization Hostage, recently established in the USA, is an independent charity that provides pastoral care and practical support to hostages and their families, during and after a kidnap. It has shown that families will often need a very fast response to be confident that their anxieties will be addressed. They recommend that this key contact needs to be available to families 24/7, and the reliability of this contact is vital to establish a trusting relationship. Hostage provides a range of professional support services and expert advice to individuals and families of kidnap victims and freed hostages. Please see the end of the book for the website and contact details.

Families want information *above all else*. They're engaged in a process of attempting to make sense of the situation their family member is in and predicting outcomes. So they will seek to absorb as much information as possible in order to make those judgements. In a world that is so reliant on the media, social networking, and other virtual communication, information can be accessed from a variety of sources, many of which are of dubious provenance with the potential to misinform, confuse, and raise unnecessary anxiety. So organizations need to be ready and able to present as much information as is possible to the family. There may be areas that cannot be discussed for reasons of operational security, but it is very likely that the family will identify what those areas are if attempts are made to evade or hide information. A far better tactic is to be honest with the family and explain what can and cannot be disclosed, with an explanation and rationale as to why this is the case.

Individuals and families also want is to know that the problem is being dealt with at the very highest level of the organization. So the family's point of contact needs to be able to demonstrate that he or she has this level of access. We'd recommend that organizations bring in someone at a senior level to reassure families that the organization is taking responsibility and action. Whoever that senior person is, he or she needs to be aware of his or her responsibilities and the potential pitfalls when communicating with a family.

What are the characteristics that make for good and effective family support? Whoever provides that support needs to be consistent, reliable, and, above all, resilient. Supporting individuals and families exposed to the trauma of having a family member abducted and held hostage has the potential to be an emotionally challenging experience. The individual or individuals providing such support will be exposed to a wide range of emotions, whatever the mode and transmission of communication. In addition, they will be dealing, albeit second-hand, with chaotic and potentially violent situations with no guarantee of satisfactory outcome.

They also need to be able to provide practical help wherever possible. It can be the little things that cause families further stress and anxiety. Having a family member kidnapped may throw up all sorts of odd and seemingly petty situations (e.g. an inability to access bank accounts/savings, if the car insurance is in the name of the kidnapped party then a road-traffic collision may lead to an impasse, or families talking to their insurance and banks call-centres find out that there isn't a drop-down box for 'policy or account-holder kidnapped'). Organizations need to be aware that it is sometimes small, previously routine things that affect a family's equilibrium. So consideration of what can be done to help with the little things will pay dividends in terms of trust.

Accessing specialist support

It is understandable and normal that returning hostages or the families affected by their abduction will experience a range of reactions characteristic of post-traumatic stress. Therefore, it is important that these reactions be seen as normal in the context of their experience. Some indeed may go on to develop trauma symptoms, which may benefit from formal therapy at some stage, but the approach in the early stages needs to takes account of the individual's and family's natural resilience and existing social and emotional resources wherever possible. Individual and family reactions vary depending on a range of factors (e.g. previous coping strategies when faced with extreme stressors or crisis, the cohesion of the family network, pre-existing vulnerabilities, the nature and method of the abduction, the length of time the relative has been held in captivity, the media attention, and, of course, whether or not the abduction ends in the murder of the relative). In addition, the publicity generated by the kidnap and the impact this has on the world stage, as in the case of some of the high-profile abductions, will also have an enormous influence on the reactions of the families.

Returning hostages will also display a range of reactions dependent on their idiosyncratic experiences. Some of these have been mentioned earlier, but factors such as the way they have been treated whilst being held hostage, exposure to significant subjective life threat whilst in captivity, experiencing torture, and long periods of isolation and deprivation will play a significant part in determining their reactions following release. Above all, it should be noted that information, advice, and guidance is important in the early stages with families and that this should be structured and consistent. Therapists providing this support should be experienced in acute presentations of trauma and crisis and working with traumatic bereavement. The main focus with families and individual family members should be based on *structured social support* (see Chapter 4) rather than conventional trauma-focused therapy, whatever the psychotherapeutic orientation of the therapist. Studies on coping with trauma have also found that problem-solving strategies and finding meaning in the traumatic event are associated with the absence of longer-term trauma symptoms and post-traumatic stress disorder. Therefore, an approach that considers these pragmatic therapeutic strategies is likely to be the most effective.

◆ **Health needs**—returning hostages who may have been held in challenging physical conditions may benefit from a comprehensive medical check-up and appropriate psychological support if indicated.

◆ **Media advice**—management of the media is often a requirement for families going through a kidnap experience and can be one of its most stressful facets. Families may well receive conflicting advice as to the stance they take to the media, whether to maintain silence or speak out publicly about their situation.

◆ **Financial advice**—a kidnap crisis can put financial pressure on a family, particularly if the main breadwinner has been taken hostage. The organization Hostage can help to explain the situation to the Inland Revenue, banks, insurance companies, and other financial institutions to ensure that they respond in the most sympathetic way possible. It is acknowledged that payment of ransoms in some circumstances is illegal, and families will be advised of this. However, an organization like Hostage does not take a stance on the ethical question of payment beyond the legalities and, recognizing that families have very difficult decisions to make, it provides support from a non-judgemental position.

Support for children

Children and adults have differing needs during and after a kidnap. Parents are often concerned to shield younger children from what is happening, which can sometimes have a negative impact if it leaves them feeling excluded. Adolescents and teenagers often struggling with their own normal developmental challenges can feel overwhelmed by what's happening, and it can be difficult for everyone to adjust when the hostage returns home. In cases such as this, specialist trauma therapists will be able to guide parents through the challenges they may face with handling their children's reactions to a variety of stressors, such as watching repeated news coverage.

Conclusions

In summary, we know that being taken hostage can have serious psychological effects. As such, it is recommended that assistance be offered on release, along with regular follow-ups to ensure that specialist treatment is available if needed, and that the individuals are managing as best they can to re-engage with their normal life. But it is the families that are most likely to require support throughout the hostage situation and afterwards. Again, depending on individual circumstances, many issues discussed in Chapter 4 (Traumatic bereavement) are relevant and significant.

Reference

Rudge, P., and Regel, S. (2014). Taken hostage. *Counselling at Work Autumn*, 9–13.

6

Medically related trauma

⊃ Key Points

- Post-traumatic symptoms and post-traumatic stress disorder (PTSD) often present following medical procedures and illnesses.

- Research has shown that post-traumatic stress can result from accidental injury, burn trauma, cancer, and other life-threatening conditions.

- Experiences of childbirth can also lead to post-traumatic symptoms and PTSD.

- Negative biological, behavioural, psychodynamic, social-cognitive, and integrative theories are reviewed.

- Medically related trauma is different from other kinds of trauma because of ongoing complications, repeated surgery, and other invasive procedures.

The prevalence of trauma and PTSD in medical settings

Having considered the epidemiology and prevalence of post-traumatic stress in a wider context, we will now focus on the specific prevalence of trauma and PTSD in medical settings. In addition, PTSD symptoms have also been described after medical illness and treatment (e.g. among cardiac arrest survivors, in general surgical units, in stroke patients, following a diagnosis of breast cancer, and after childbirth). This chapter presents an overview of some of the likely and perhaps less obvious areas where post-traumatic stress may present, either on its own or as part of a broader picture of psychological distress.

In the chapter, we also look at the impact of physical injuries following industrial accidents and road-traffic collisions. There are also some suggestions offered as to how some longer term psychological difficulties may be avoided by adopting some relatively simple strategies at an early stage.

Modern medicine often uses invasive procedures, for which most individuals have little real preparation or understanding. Health professionals are not infallible, and mistakes and accidents unfortunately can, and do, occur during medical procedures. A complication occurring during a procedure, or a medical accident, can have profound effects upon the individual. In addition to the trauma and shock that a complication or error has caused, patients also have to contend with the fact that the very people who they felt were there to help them have played a role in their distress. This can give rise to feelings of helplessness and uncontrollability, as well as a future loss of trust in health professionals, distrust of future diagnosis and advice, and fear of future treatments. Some researchers have concluded that post-traumatic stress is prolonged after medical events, presumably, in part, because the affected individual is unable to control the situation. Rates will also vary depending on a variety of factors, but mostly these will be due to the nature and type of the stressor (e.g. whether the illness or injury was the result of a burn trauma, obstetric/gynaecological procedures, an RTC, or some other life-threatening illness, such as a stroke).

🕮 Fay's story

Fay, age 47, underwent a planned admission to a surgical ward to undergo a hysterectomy. She had been an inpatient previously, and as such, she found all of the staff she encountered to be helpful and supportive and she was left with a positive view of 'hospitals'. Consequently, she had a positive outlook before her admission for a hysterectomy. Unfortunately, during the operation, problems occurred, resulting in her being admitted to an intensive care unit (ICU) for 6 days, following which she developed an infection requiring a total hospital stay in excess of 3 weeks. Fay felt that the staff on the ward that she went to from the ICU treated her unsympathetically, in that she believed that they thought she was 'overreacting' about the amount of pain and discomfort she was experiencing. Her symptoms included flashbacks, nightmares, avoidance of hospitals (and of all media triggers concerning medical matters), a sense of foreshortened future (feelings that her life may somehow be cut short), and a high level of irritability/anger.

Road-traffic collisions

The most common presentation in trauma and orthopaedic units will be those arising from a variety of accidental injuries, ranging from road-traffic collisions (RTCs) to industrial accidents. Department of Transport (2015) data from the UK show that there were 1,775 reported road deaths in 2014, an increase of 4% compared with 2013. The 1,775 road deaths in 2014 comprise the third-lowest annual total on record after 2012 and 2013. There were 45% fewer fatalities in 2014 than in 2005. Pedestrians accounted for three-quarters of the increase in fatalities between 2013 and 2014. Pedestrian fatalities increased by 12% from 398 in 2013 to 446 in 2014. In 2014, car occupants accounted for 45% of road deaths; pedestrians 25%; motorcyclists 19%; and cyclists 6%. In 2014, there were 22,807 seriously injured casualties in reported RTCs. This represents a 5.3% rise from 2013, but it is lower than the 23,039 seriously injured in 2012. There were 194,477 casualties of all severities in reported RTCs during 2014. This is the second-lowest level on record, although it is 5.9% higher than in 2013. It is the first increase in overall casualties in a decade.

The number of cyclist fatalities has remained between 104 and 118 since 2008. In 2014, there were 113 deaths, up 4 deaths from the 2013 figures. This change is not part of a meaningful trend and is not statistically significant. However, there was an 8.2% rise in the number of seriously injured cyclists to 3,401 in 2014. With the exception of 2012 to 2013, the number of seriously injured pedal cyclists has increased every year since the low of 2,174 in 2004. This long-term rise indicates that there is an ever-increasing problem with cyclist casualties.

The range of RTC survivors includes pedestrians, motorcyclists, and cyclists. However, the research literature on RTCs has tended to focus on motor vehicle accidents per se. The rates for PTSD following RTCs vary from 11% to 46%. In a study of a consecutive series of 188 RTC victims, a quarter described long-term psychiatric consequences of three overlapping types:

◆ Mood disorder

◆ PTSD

◆ Phobic anxiety about travel

In addition, a fifth of people complained of persistent and disabling anxiety. One-fifth of the sample with major or minor injuries experienced severe initial distress, characterized by altered mood and horrific memories. Nineteen of the sample (11%) met the criteria for PTSD at 1 year (Mayou, Bryant, and Duthie, 1993).

📖 Michaela's story

Michaela is a 28-year-old professional woman who was admitted following a serious RTC and has suffered severe multiple injuries. She had stopped on the motorway to help at an accident. She saw another driver running towards her waving at her to stop and help. As she stopped on the hard shoulder and was preparing to get out of out of the car, her car and the other driver were hit by a lorry travelling at speed, which could not stop in time. The other man was killed instantly, and she was trapped in the car and had to be cut out by the emergency services. After 3 weeks in hospital, she was having tearful episodes, experiencing problems sleeping (unrelated to pain), was low in mood, and was expressing feelings of guilt at having survived when someone else had died. When originally offered help by the ward staff, she had declined, but then later requested to be seen.

She was given the opportunity to discuss the circumstances of the accident (which she had previously not done in any depth for fear of upsetting her relatives), her thoughts and emotional reactions at the time, and her current difficulties and reactions (e.g. her guilt feelings). She also expressed her anxieties about what she had been told by friends and relatives about the accident, as she had a poor memory of events. As a consequence, she had formed her own narrative based on what she'd been told, thus she had 'reconstructed' memories, some of which were inaccurate, as confirmed by the police and eyewitnesses. The issue of 'reconstructed memory' was discussed in some depth, and she was able to develop a more accurate narrative, which helped her deal with the guilt she had been feeling over the death of the other driver. She was provided with education, advice, and guidance, as described above, and encouraged to ask questions about her reactions and responses. Her reactions were normalized in the context of her experience. She was later seen once on the ward for follow-up and then in the outpatient department. Six months later, she was making a good recovery with no psychological ill effects. She reported that the early session and the follow-up had helped make sense of her feelings and reactions at the time and in the subsequent days and weeks.

Coping with the effects of traumatic injury

Physical injury following accidents, such as RTCs, can be classed as one of the 'complicating' factors that we looked at in earlier chapters. The reason for this is that such injuries, often regardless of their magnitude, can have an impact upon psychological recovery. This often happens because of the repeated visits to hospital for surgery, physiotherapy, and other treatments. For example, following a burn trauma, the patient may have repeated appointments for surgery for skin grafting and correction of previous surgery. It can also have an impact upon work and employment prospects and inevitably affect levels of social and leisure activity. Previously, avoidance following traumatic events has been noted to be common but it leads to problems in the longer term if not monitored and dealt with gradually and systematically over time. However, with individuals who have suffered a physical injury, there is often an 'enforced avoidance' because of practical reasons, which can lead to further problems later. For example, the person may have had a severe leg injury, which would inhibit their levels of physical activity and mobility and, consequently, would have to forego many activities he or she would previously have undertaken, for the simple reason of being physically unable to carry them out. This 'enforced avoidance' may often lead to a gradual reduction of social contact and, therefore, a reduction of social support, leading to the development of symptoms, such as mental and behavioural avoidance and the reduction of confidence, self-esteem, and mood. This then feeds back into the cycle of a loss of routine and inactivity, and a reduction of social contact, and eventually becomes a very difficult pattern to break. There are some useful strategies in the wake of being exposed to a traumatic injury. By this, we mean injuries that have been sustained in circumstances that are sudden, unexpected, often violent, and sometimes life-threatening. Examples would be RTCs, industrial accidents, workplace violence, and transportation accidents, which may involve multiple fractures, serious lacerations, and amputations.

Some useful strategies

◆ Try to establish a routine as soon as possible—when you get home from hospital, try and consider ways in which you can be active, however small at first, during the day and through the week.

◆ Draw up an activity schedule for each week and, if necessary, break each day into 1-hour time slots.

◆ Don't be over-ambitious at the start, pace yourself; a little is better than too much—don't set yourself up to fail.

◆ Try not to sleep during the day—this can be difficult, but planning activities would help.

◆ Try to keep a sleep diary and ask others to help you with this, noting your sleep patterns, wherever possible.

◆ With regard to activity—think of things you used to like doing but are not able to do now—is it possible to try some of these activities in a small way given your limitations?

◆ Think of things you have perhaps always wanted to do or learn about but have never had the time to try—this might be a good opportunity to ask somebody to get you information from the library or other sources in order to try and acquire new knowledge or perhaps a skill, if that is possible.

◆ Try to incorporate the activities into a schedule for the week.

◆ Be practical, don't overdo it. Start with 10–15-minute periods—don't attempt activities for unreasonably long periods (e.g. an hour or more). You may find you become tired quite soon, have to give up the activity, and then either blame yourself or find it difficult to return and continue where you left off.

- Try to be consistent.

- Remember, it is better to do something for a brief period than do nothing at all!

- Activity has a positive effect on mood over time.

Burn trauma

Within the last decade, there has been an emerging interest in the complex nature of post-traumatic symptoms and PTSD following burn injury. There is evidence that post-traumatic symptoms and PTSD are not uncommon in burn survivors. In the UK, about 500 deaths per year occur as a result of injury by fire, and over 28,000 persons suffer serious injuries. In the USA, it is estimated that approximately 1% annually of the population sustains burns (i.e. approximately 300,000 people, of whom 7000 die) (Neophytos et al. 2016). It would be hardly surprising if burn injury, which is a painful, frightening, and extraordinary traumatic event, precipitated post-traumatic symptoms in some burns survivors. Other risk and vulnerability factors found to be important were age, social class, and whether individuals lived on their own or with a large family, pointing to the importance, again, of social support. There is also no clear relationship between where the injury occurs on the body and the frequency and severity of psychological side effects.

Turner, Thompson and Rossers (1995) research with some of the most severely physically damaged survivors of the 1987 King's Cross Fire showed that many were troubled by nightmares (invariably involving flames); all described a heightened sense of vigilance in everyday situations (e.g. crossing the road). They also experienced an intense sense of the frailty of human life and an expectation of further disasters. Many reported flashbacks, disturbed sleep, avoidance of common activities, and emotional difficulties on the anniversary of the disaster—all symptoms characteristic of PTSD.

The lesson to be learned here, as the authors of the study concluded, is that:

> . . . early psychological contact is vital for the emotional and physical well-being of the patient in the early stages of recovery.

The development of PTSD in children post burn has also been studied. Bakker and colleagues (2013) found that when compared with other clinical samples of children, children who suffered burn trauma had especially high levels of psychiatric disturbance, including PTSD. Some believe that the burn treatment itself becomes a traumatic event and that for some children, the longer hospitalization is extended, with the daily cycle of dressing changes and physiotherapy, the more regressed and withdrawn they become.

📄 Jane and Robert's story

Jane, age 29, and her 2-year-old son, Robert, were the survivors of an explosion that occurred in the family home. The accident occurred a few days before Christmas. Jane was also 3-months pregnant at the time. The boiler exploded, virtually demolishing the living room and causing severe damage estimated at £12,000.

Robert was seriously injured, suffering a depressed fracture of the frontal lobe of the brain and 12% burns, which required grafting, with the areas of most concern being his right forehead (the eyebrow being missing) and the right side of his torso. Jane sustained burns to both legs, mostly superficial. She also received a head injury, sustained when she was hit by flying debris. Both mother and son were taken to the local A&E department and then admitted to the burns unit. Her unborn child was unharmed.

After the accident, she suffered from depression and experienced a variety of symptoms, which met the diagnostic criteria for PTSD. She was unable to discuss her son's injuries (which were severe) or her own. She would avoid television programmes and magazine or newspaper articles containing material that reminded her of the accident. She was experiencing panic attacks and bouts of irritability and exhibiting obsessional behaviour, resulting in frequent checking of electrical appliances, such as the gas fire and the cooker.

Her relationship with her husband was also under considerable strain, and she found that she was becoming overprotective and over concerned with her son's welfare, the latter inevitably having implications for his future psychological development and well-being. Jane was unable to discuss the accident with anybody she might meet on a casual or social basis; she would become extremely distressed and withdraw from the situation. Jane was also experiencing bouts of anxiety triggered by the continuing treatment Robert required because of his injuries. Jane also had marked concern about Robert's ability to integrate with other children, owing to the cosmetic nature of his injuries, and worried lest this caused problems at school and in later life; to some extent, her concerns were not without substance.

Jane also experienced feelings of guilt and anger about the incident and her part in Robert's aftercare. She felt that she could have done more at the time of the accident to help to remove him from the scene of the explosion. She recalled that at the time of the accident, she made every attempt to try to reach her son, but was so bewildered, shocked, and

> frightened that she could not locate him, as the room was in darkness and she was also handicapped by her own injuries. Consequently, she made for the nearest chink of light and stumbled free to get help. She began to see this as an act of selfishness rather than the only course of action open to her at the time.

Jane received 12 sessions of cognitive-behavioural therapy (CBT) and was able to make a good recovery and develop new perspectives and coping strategies. Her recovery had a positive effect on Robert, who was able to integrate well with other children, often being overheard by teachers at school discussing his experiences, both of the accident and at hospital, with the other children in a positive way.

> Even if you are badly hurt, the doctors and nurses at the hospital are great! They can make things better most of the time ... and they have loads of great DVDS!

PTSD resulting from obstetric trauma

Studies from various countries suggest a prevalence of between 0 and 7% of women fulfilling diagnostic criteria for PTSD at some point after giving birth (Menage 1993). Prevalence rates are higher in at-risk groups, such as women who have a premature or stillbirth, with reports of up to 26%. Cross-cultural comparison of prevalence rates suggests similar prevalence in Europe (i.e. Sweden, Italy, UK, and The Netherlands), the USA, and Australia.

The available evidence seems to suggest that the prevalence of PTSD in women after birth in developed countries is approximately 1%–2% (Ayers et al. 2008).

In a review by Ballard, Stanley, and Brockington (1995) of 500 women's experiences of obstetric and gynaecological procedures, over a 100 described their experiences as being 'very distressing' or 'terrifying'. Of these women, at follow-up, 30 of them met the criteria for PTSD. These women identified that they experienced feelings of powerlessness during the procedure, a lack of information as to the procedures taking place, the experience of physical pain, and a perceived 'unsympathetic' attitude on the part of the staff.

Research has described PTSD resulting from obstetric trauma where the labour was medically complicated, painful, prolonged, and threatening to the life of the mother and the baby. Another study by Wijma, Soderquist, and Wijma (1997), into childbirth experiences in Sweden, found post-traumatic stress reactions after emergency Caesarean sections. Of 25 women interviewed a few days and a few months after emergency section, 19 had experienced their delivery as a traumatic event, but, after 2 months, none of the women met the criteria of PTSD. However, 13 women had various forms of post-traumatic stress reactions, and some of these had high levels of intrusive thoughts.

📖 Jan's story

Jan was a 31-year-old mother of two who was having her third child. She began having contractions earlier than anticipated, which eventually resulted in her being taken to hospital. As she was staying with friends for the weekend, in another city, she was taken to a hospital she did not know. She developed unexpected complications and, during delivery in the labour suite, she suffered a significant loss of blood. She recalled a lot of doctors and midwives being present, a lot of noise and activity, and then, as she was drifting in and out of consciousness, she heard a male voice saying, 'I think we are losing her . . .'—she wasn't sure if this meant her or the baby, as both she and her partner knew that it was a girl. Soon after, she lost consciousness, and when she woke in the antenatal unit the following day, she felt disorientated, her surroundings felt strange and unreal, and she was convinced that she had died. She gradually realized this wasn't the case when she saw her daughter beside her.

Nevertheless, the experience left her with marked post-traumatic reactions, which later developed into significant symptoms of PTSD. She did not understand what was happening to her and why she was feeling the way she was. This very much echoes Laura's story earlier. As is often usual, she began to avoid thinking and talking about her experience, which subsequently led to other avoidances, such as crossing the street when she saw a mother and baby, not reading newspaper or magazine articles about pregnancy and childbirth, and switching off the TV or changing channels if she saw programmes that had a resonance to her experience.

Conclusion

The experience of traumatic events often results in the shattering of basic assumptions that the victims hold about themselves, others, and the world. It is common for this to occur after a traumatic injury or traumatic experiences resulting from medical procedures. There are three basic assumptions about the self, others, and the world that are commonly shared by most people. We may not be aware of these, but they are often related to the following:

- The belief in personal invulnerability (i.e. nothing is going to happen to us);

- The perception of the world as meaningful and comprehensible (i.e. generally there is a predictability to our lives); and

- The view of self and others in a positive light.

Therefore, the assessment of attribution and meaning is vital in understanding an individual's reactions following traumatic events. Traumatic events have the potential to shatter these basic assumptions. The relevance of shattered assumptions and the significance of anger are worth bearing in mind. Anger is a common emotional reaction in victims of trauma. However, it can also prove to be an extremely debilitating emotion. It often focuses on the lack of concern or apology from those believed to be responsible and the lack of recognition of the suffering and disability caused.

Some of this distress can be diffused by a simple, straightforward explanation of their difficulties and to be told that they are responding in a normal way to a distressing experience, and told what course their symptoms may take (i.e. that the majority of individuals return to normal emotional functioning within a few days/weeks).

References

Ayers, S., Joseph, S., McKenzie-McHarg, K., Slade, P., and Wijma, K. (2008). Post-traumatic stress following childbirth: current issues and recommendations for future research. *Journal of Psychosomatic Obstetrics and Gynaecology* 29, 240–250

Bakker, A., Maertens, K. J., Van Son, M. J., Van Loey, N. E. (2013). Psychological consequences of pediatric burns from a child and family perspective: a review of the empirical literature. *Clinical Psychology Review.* 33, 361–371.

Ballard, C. G., Stanley, A. K., and Brockington, I. F. (1995). Post-traumatic stress disorder (PTSD) after childbirth. *British Journal of Psychiatry* 166, 525–528.

Department for Transport. (2015). Reported road casualties in Great Britain 2014. Statistical release 2015. Department for Transport. https://www.gov.uk/government/uploads/system/uploads/attachment_data/file/438040/reported-road-casualties-in-great-britain-main-results-2014-release.pdf. [Accessed 1 June 2016].

Menage, J. (1993). Post-traumatic stress disorder in women who have undergone obstetric and/or gynaecological procedures. *Journal of Reproductive & Infant Psychology* 11, 221–228.

Mayou, R., Bryant, B., and Duthie, R. (1993). Psychiatric consequences of road traffic accidents. *British Medical Journal* 307(6905), 647–651.

Neophytos, S., Buchan, I., and Dunn, K. W. (2016). A review of the international Burn Injury Database (iBID) for England and Wales: descriptive analysis of burn injuries 2003-2011. BMJOpen 2015;5:e006184. doi:10.1136/bmjopen-2014-006184. [Accessed 1 June 2016].

Turner, S. W., Thompson, J., and Rosser, R. M. (1995). The Kings Cross Fire: psychological reactions. *Journal of Traumatic Stress* 8(3), 419–427.

Wijma, K., Soderquist, J., and Wijma, B. (1997). Post traumatic stress after childbirth: a cross sectional study. *Journal of Anxiety Disorders* 11(6), 587–597.

7

Cultural responses to trauma

➔ Key Points

- Currently we are living through the most significant refugee crisis since the Second World War as result of the conflict in Syria and the enduring legacy of the conflicts in Iraq and Afghanistan.

- Cultural responses to trauma and loss vary depending on age, ethnic differences, and gender.

- Within different cultures, post-traumatic stress disorder (PTSD) may not always appear to be appropriate as a diagnosis.

- It is possible to adapt different therapies to work with refugees and survivors of torture, but this needs to be considered alongside other community-based approaches.

- Humanitarian aid agencies are developing psychosocial programmes to cater to the needs of individuals, families, and communities affected by complex emergencies, such as natural disasters and civil conflict.

- Psychosocial programmes are designed to promote and enhance the natural resilience of populations affected by complex emergencies.

Introduction

In previous chapters we've discussed common responses to trauma and considerations that need to be taken into account to understand individual, family, and community responses. However, responses to traumatic events in different cultures are often complex, and psychological reactions will vary depending on age, cultural and ethnic differences, and gender. In addition, the notion of psychotherapy or counselling will often be an alien concept as access to 'talking therapies' are rare, and many cultures would turn to traditional healers. However, this will be covered later in the chapter. The awareness of the impact of traumatic events on different cultures and societies has become widespread in an age where advances in communication technologies mean that the human costs following conflict, disasters, and other emergencies are brought into our lives, not only through the media of television but also through readily available access to the Internet. It is beyond the scope of this book to examine cultural responses in significant depth, but the intention here is to give an overview of cultural factors that may influence and affect individual and community experiences of traumatic events.

Currently we are living through the most significant refugee crisis since the Second World War as result of the conflict in Syria and the enduring legacy of the conflicts in Iraq and Afghanistan. The United Nations High Commissioner for Refugees (UNHCR, 2016a) has described Europe as living through a 'maritime refugee crisis' of historic proportions. It asserts that the majority of migrants taking the sea route are eligible for protection. In the first half of 2015, 43,900 Syrians arrived in Western Europe by sea, and the UNHCR (2016b) observed that in 2014, 95% Syrians after arrival were acknowledged in Europe as refugees. The European Agency for the Management of Operational Co-operation at the External Borders of the Member States of the European Union (Frontex) estimated that in 2012, 15,151 migrants travelled across the central Mediterranean. These numbers grew to 45,298 in 2013 and then 170,664 in 2014 (Frontex 2015). The UNHCR also reported that in April 2015, 1,308 refugees and migrants drowned or went missing in a single month. Of the worlds' refugees, the UNHCR (2016c) estimates that 51% were under the age of 18, the highest figure in over a decade. Inevitably, there are significant implications for the impact of trauma in these populations.

In the chapter, first, the impact of trauma on refugees is discussed, and then there is an overview of what humanitarian aid organizations are currently doing to address the needs of populations affected by conflict, disaster, and what are often described as 'complex emergencies'. These are situations where one humanitarian disaster or catastrophe is affected by another, such as in Sri Lanka and Aceh in Indonesia, where the impact of the Tsunami and relief efforts were complicated by many years of civil conflict in the affected areas.

The concept of psychological trauma and cultural differences across cultures

Across cultures, people differ in what they believe and understand about life and death, what they feel, what elicits those feelings, the perceived implications of those feelings, their expression, and the appropriateness of certain feelings and strategies for dealing with feelings that cannot be directly expressed. A cross-cultural perspective demonstrates the variety, for example, in people's responses to death and dying, and the process of mourning. Rather than being process-orientated, mourning is seen as an adaptive response to specific task demands arising from loss that must be dealt with regardless of individual, culture, or historical era. Stroebe (1992) challenged the belief in the importance of 'grief work' for adjustment to bereavement. She examined claims made in theoretical formulations and principles of grief counselling and therapy concerning the necessity of working through loss. Grief reactions are also patterned by the culture, formed by one's society's belief systems and expectations and values and norms for relationships and bonds. This will influence both expression and duration of grief reactions across different cultural settings. In essence, sensitivity to the culturally appropriate needs for ritual, in responding to grief and providing for privacy and personal needs, are paramount.

Research on post-traumatic reactions in non-Western groups has mostly been conducted in Western Europe and the USA to meet the needs of refugees from developing countries. Differences in the prevalence of PTSD across ethnic and cultural groups have been reported. However, there are several problematic issues related to cross-cultural trauma research. One of the reasons for discrepancies in cross-cultural studies is that Western diagnostic criteria are not always applicable in non-Western cultures, and the diagnosis of PTSD has been controversial.

For example, a recent study on Tibetan refugees in India demonstrated that in this population, the destruction of religious symbols was a major stressor (Terheggen et al. 2001). If culturally defined stressors were not heeded, the amount of stress experienced would be evaluated lower than it actually was. The same group of workers also noted that some symptoms common to trauma survivors, such as guilt, were displayed far less than would be expected, explained by the fact that the word *guilt* does not even have a Tibetan equivalent. A further illustration can be seen in the above-mentioned study within a religious context. Buddhism implies that 'hopelessness lies in the nature of the world'. The acknowledgement of the all-pervasive presence of suffering in the world is almost 'endorsed' by Buddhism. A 'non-disorder' frame of reference for 'depressive' symptoms is therefore present within Buddhist cultures. A recent study that attempted to assess PTSD in a radically non-Western culture, that of Kalahari Bushmen, found that the results compared closely with PTSD assessments in other non-Western societies (McCall and Resick 2003).

There have been a number of studies conducted with survivors of torture and political violence, which have shown that the most common symptoms displayed across the cultures sampled were those associated with the diagnoses of depression, anxiety disorders, and PTSD. They manifest themselves in different ways within cultures, but the symptoms tend to fit the general diagnostic criteria for the disorders mentioned previously. Some individuals will also have suffered multiple losses, in addition to their torture experiences.

Definition of torture

In 1984, the United Nations, in the Convention against Torture and Other Cruel, Inhuman or Degrading Treatment or Punishment, adopted the following definition:

> For the purpose of this Convention, the term 'torture' means any act by which severe pain or suffering, whether physical or mental, is intentionally inflicted on a person for such purpose as obtaining from him or a third person information or a confession, punishing him for an act he or a third person has committed, or is suspected of having committed, or intimidating or coercing him or a third person, or for any reason based on discrimination of any kind, when such pain or suffering is inflicted by, or at the instigation of, or with the consent or acquiescence of, a public official or other person acting in an official capacity. It does not include pain or suffering arising only from, inherent in or incidental to lawful sanctions.

> Text extract from *Inhuman or Degrading Treatment or Punishment* by United Nations Humans Rights Office, Convention against Torture and Other Cruel (OHCHR), Copyright © United Nations 1984. Reprinted with the permission of the United Nations.

This definition was restricted to apply only to nations and to government-sponsored torture. It did not include cases of countries where torture, such as mutilation or whipping, are practices of lawful punishment, nor did it include cases of torture practised by gangs or hate groups. In 1986, the World Health Organization (WHO) working group introduced the concept of Organized Violence, which was defined as:

> The inter-human infliction of significant, avoidable pain and suffering by an organized group according to a declared or implied strategy and/or system of ideas and attitudes. It comprises any violent action that is unacceptable by general human standards, and relates to the victim's feelings. Organized violence includes 'torture, cruel inhuman or degrading treatment or punishment' as in Article 5 of the United Nations Universal Declaration of Human Rights (1948). Imprisonment without trial, mock executions, hostage-taking, or any other form of violent deprivation of liberty, also falls under the heading of organized violence.

> Text extract from World Health Organization, *Considering conflict. Concept paper for first Health as a Bridge for Peace, Consultative Meeting,* Copyright © 1997. Reprinted with the permission of the World Health Organization.

Torture is a complex trauma that often occurs within the context of widespread persecution and human rights violations. Furthermore, the nature of modern armed conflict is such that whole populations are at risk of suffering extensive trauma, losses, injustices, and displacement. The estimates of the numbers of asylum seekers who have been victims of torture or organized violence vary considerably, depending on their country of origin and definitions used. The UNHCR estimated:

◆ In 2014, the total number of refugees and others of concern forcibly displaced worldwide numbered 59.5 million.

◆ There are 38.2 million internally displaced people (IDP) worldwide, equal to approximately 33,000 per day.

◆ Almost half of the world's forcibly displaced people are children and many spend their entire childhood far from home. Whether they are refugees, IDP, asylum seekers, or stateless, children are at a greater risk of abuse, neglect, violence, exploitation, trafficking, or forced military recruitment. They may also have witnessed or experienced violent acts and/or been separated from their families.

◆ At the end of 2014, the UNHCR was caring for approximately 32.3 million IDP worldwide.

◆ The Democratic Republic of the Congo, Iraq, Nigeria, South Sudan, and Syria account for 60% of new displacement worldwide (UNHCR 2016c).

Assessment of trauma across cultures

The massive trauma experienced by refugees and torture victims raises ethical and clinical questions about the potential negative impact upon them of using checklists or questionnaires, as have previously been described. Secondly, the diverse ethnocultural and political backgrounds require assessment questionnaires sensitive to a wide range of traumatic events and experiences. For example, the traumatic experiences of Chilean political prisoners were dramatically different to those of Indo-Chinese refugees. Finally, while specific symptoms have been clearly linked to the trauma of torture, the DSM-V criterion for PTSD has not been established as a valid disease construct in non-Western cultures. Cross-national comparisons by the WHO suggest that, despite core features of major depression, each culture has its own specific symptoms. PTSD criteria may reveal a similar pattern across cultures; however, a central universal core of PTSD remains to be established. There are issues concerning the definition and nature of traumatic stressors in different cultures. These are often different depending on the cultural settings. Therefore, a standardized checklist could under- or overestimate the prevalence of traumatic stressors, if the list were not sensitive to the cultural values of the population studied.

Nevertheless, there have been a number of studies conducted with disaster survivors, refugees, and survivors of torture and political violence, which used the most culturally appropriate assessment methods available. It would appear that the most common symptoms displayed across the cultures sampled in the above-mentioned studies, were those associated with the diagnoses of depression, anxiety, and PTSD. They manifest themselves in different ways within cultures, but the symptoms tend to fit the general diagnostic criteria for the disorders mentioned herein. In recent years there have also been studies that have attempted to address the issue of assessment and the use of culturally sensitive questionnaires with some degree of success.

Recently, critics of the concept of PTSD as applied to non-Western settings have also argued that there is no evidence that mental health problems are higher in populations exposed to conflict and other complex emergencies, citing Northern Ireland as one such example. Critics further suggest that over the last 30 years of civil conflict, there has been little evidence of significant impact on referral rates to mental health services. However, a recent published community survey to assess the effects of the civil unrest (the Troubles, as they have come to be colloquially known) on the general population concluded that exposure to the Troubles has resulted in a significant and independent detrimental effect on the mental health of the population in Northern Ireland. Within the context of the Northern Ireland 'Troubles', we are drawn to the observations of Arlene Healy, Consultant Family Therapist and former Head of the Family Trauma Centre in Belfast, who has written eloquently about the 'context of silence' in Northern Ireland. When discussing her work with children and families affected by the 'Troubles', she provides an explanation for the perceived lack of mental health problems within the population of the province.

Healy discusses the context of silence that has existed for over 30 years: silence from those involved and from social services, silence within higher education establishments and those involved in the education and training of health and social care professionals, and silence amongst those planning health and social care provision in the province.

She has argued that finding a language adequately explaining the impact of trauma on families was difficult because of the vacuum of silence that surrounded decades of violence in which a language to discuss such traumatic events failed to develop. By 1994, the peace process had gained momentum, and a sense of hope was growing—it began to be easier to discuss the impact of the Troubles. Society in Northern Ireland had also reflected this change, including this newly found sense of hope, through the media and in literature. The establishment of a Victims Commission in 1998, following the publication of the Bloomfield report, led to the setting up of a Family Trauma Centre in 1999, a province-wide service. Furthermore, there has been the establishment of Trauma Advisory Panels in Northern Ireland—a clear acceptance that the mental health needs of the population in relation to their traumatic experiences warrant addressing. In addition, the Cost of the Troubles Study concluded that 30% of those who participated in and had been exposed to violence associated with the Troubles had needs approximating to PTSD and related conditions. These factors were further supported in a recent review of mental health and learning disability in Northern Ireland, validating the view that psychological trauma had not been sufficiently addressed as a specific health issue.

Factors affecting asylum seekers and refugees

Health and mental health practitioners are accustomed to seeing culturally diverse populations in their regular practice. Inevitably, many will be refugees who are survivors of torture and organized violence. Whilst not all will experience such extremes of traumatic events, these particular individuals often present to therapists with complex psychotherapeutic challenges. For many there will be normal and understandable problems of adjustment to a new culture and society, combined with the practical problems presented by the host country's asylum processes and procedures. There will be no attempt to describe these laws and processes here, as they vary considerably from country to country and are often subject to frequent changes influenced by national priorities and international events. Universally, those fleeing wars or religious or ethnic persecution were once referred to collectively as refugees. However, over the last decade, the term *asylum seeker* has been adopted and used by almost all EU countries. Essentially, this means the same thing in these countries, that is, those seeking a safe haven are given the status of 'asylum seekers' until their cases have been heard and they are given the right to stay in the country, whereby they are then given 'refugee' status and are usually able to access rights and benefits available to citizens of the host country. One common factor pertinent to all asylum seekers is the inability to seek or obtain paid employment before they are granted refugee status. This inevitably has significant implications for the mental health of individuals and families, as it is well known that access to employment has a positive impact on mental health and well-being. There is also great variability in other areas, such as access to housing, healthcare, legal aid, interpreters, and other resources to improve the quality of their lives.

Where asylum seekers and refugees have been welcomed and offered opportunities to develop their potential and capacities and participate actively in the affairs of the host country, they often overcome major adversities from their past. On the other hand, where they are marginalized, victimized, and held back, they tend to become enmeshed in stereotypical roles that reinforce negative beliefs and values, leading to further persecution and repression. After periods of upheaval, most individuals and communities become proactive in efforts to re-establish their equilibrium and take steps to achieve recovery and promote well-being. Common problems experienced by those seeking asylum and by refugees are:

- A loss of identity.
- Being scapegoated by host society, often leading to isolation, hostility, violence, and racism.

- Being dependant on state benefits to survive.

- Not having adequate access to health and social care benefits.

- Experiencing high levels of psychosomatic complaints (i.e. presenting with physical problems often masking psychological difficulties).

- Problems of adjustment to the host society and local community.

- Depression.

- Anxiety, guilt, and shame.

- Symptoms of post-traumatic stress and PTSD.

By attempting to define and establish more clearly the links between types of trauma, cultural, mental, and social mechanisms and structures that influence these experiences, and the ongoing post-traumatic social environment, it may be possible to intervene early with those refugees at greatest risk of persisting psychological and social disability. It will be inevitable that refugees will often only respond to therapists who adopt an unambiguous position in supporting their human rights—an important ethical and practical consideration.

Issues relating to treatment

It is vital to establish a good rapport with the patient at the outset. An understanding of the social, cultural, and political landscape of the torture survivor is important. Giving the message that the therapist has taken time to try to understand and make sense of the circumstances that lead them to seek asylum is key to establishing a good rapport and relationship. It is also useful to try to speak a few simple words in the patient's own language, if possible. A simple greeting or welcoming phrase in the patient's own language can make a significant difference. The role of the interpreter is crucial. In many cases, the only qualification the interpreter has is the ability to speak another language. They will often have little, if any, training in mental health issues. Guidelines for therapists and interpreters are given in more detail below.

Close collaboration is recommended with other services, such as physiotherapy, which can often assist in dealing with the numerous physical problems manifested by torture survivors, such as muscular skeletal problems and the effects of other physical injuries. Linking and liaising with community resources at an early stage is vital in trying to bridge the divide between the voluntary and statutory services. It is also useful to have information on the survivors' host country and the context of their experience. The development of a 'Country File' can be a useful resource, with information being gleaned from a variety of websites (see Appendix 2). This can hold updates on the country of origin, together with previous and current political developments, historical and geographical information, human rights violations, and related information.

Knowledge and awareness of some of these issues can have a significant positive impact on the establishment of the relationship and rapport between the practitioner and torture survivor. Medication also has a place in the range of therapeutic options found effective in helping survivors. There are also clear indications that selective anti-depressants can show benefits if used appropriately in specific cases.

It is beyond the scope of this chapter to provide details of which therapies are the most effective, but many different approaches have been used, and often therapists may use a combination of approaches and strategies. Recently case reports have been published demonstrating that cognitive behavioural therapy (CBT) can be useful with survivors of torture (Regel and Berliner, 2007). Cognitive behavioural interventions also involve encouraging survivors to think that their behaviour under torture was a normal human response necessary for survival; that torture is designed to induce total loss of control and helplessness, which might explain why they behaved the way they did. Torture survivors also need to establish new values and assumptions about themselves, others, and the world that enable the development of trust, meaning, and behaviours that are more functional. However, therapy should not be seen as an activity that happens in isolation. Another extremely important aspect of treatment is the integration of the patient into the community. This involves the development of social networks and participation and involvement in meaningful psychosocial activities, such as education, employment, voluntary work (in their community), and cultural and political activities. Whilst some attempt to integrate with their local community, many find themselves socially isolated. Therefore, a holistic approach that involves the development and use of a variety of social support networks should be adopted when working with asylum seekers and refugees.

🗎 Farouq's story

Farouq was a 30-year-old male of Iraqi Kurdish origin, referred by his general practitioner (GP). He presented with low mood, suicidal thoughts, low confidence, low self-esteem, sleep difficulties, frequent nightmares, and a marked social phobia, as a result of his experiences whilst incarcerated and tortured by the security forces in Iraq under Saddam Hussein's regime. Farouq was a photographer and artist, and he became involved in the opposition movement, producing anti-government literature. He was subsequently arrested and detained for over 3 months. During that time he underwent prolonged interrogations, frequent beatings with electric cables, and dousing in cold water, and he sustained physical trauma of his genitalia as a result of physical abuse. In addition, he was also suspended off the floor for hours from a banister or from his cell windows, with his arms bent backwards, a common form of torture used by the Iraqi intelligence services. He was twice taken to hospital when he was no longer able to withstand the torture and had collapsed, only to be revived and returned to prison. He was eventually freed after 3 months and, subsequently, he fled the country to the UK. There was no previous history of psychiatric problems, and the anti-depressants from his GP had begun to have a positive effect, albeit small, on his mood. At assessment, his asylum case was ongoing, and inevitably, this presented him with further very real anxieties and uncertainties about his future.

Farouq received 12 hourly sessions of CBT, over a period of 6 months. A key focus of early sessions was education regarding the development and maintenance of his mental health problems. This was followed with a combination of graded exposure to feared situations, simple anxiety-management techniques, anti-depressant medication, and involvement with community resources and activities. Eye Movement Desensitization and Reprocessing (EMDR; see Chapter 9)was also used with Farouq, to treat the traumatic memories arising from the torture. Through early discussions, he was able to see the link between his torture experiences and his loss of confidence and self-esteem, which then led to his phobic anxiety in social situations. He was also able to make connections with regards to his symptoms and emotional responses. For example, he was given explanations as to how this pattern developed through avoidance, and this was illustrated with simple flow diagrams demonstrating cause and effect, using specific examples from his own experience.

The common reactions to torture, and this presentation in others with similar experiences, were also discussed, thus allowing him to see that his reactions were not 'abnormal'. There was also careful negotiation concerning his goals, especially to determine what would be realistic and achievable. For example, regarding the elimination of symptoms, he was encouraged to accept that in the initial phase of therapy, whilst there would very likely be a reduction in the potency or impact of the symptoms, that the aim of therapy would be to enable him to come to terms with his experience, rather than 'get over it'. He was also encouraged to identify ways in which he would know that things were improving, and these became his 'targets' (e.g. one of his targets was to be able to 'contribute to meetings and activities at the refugee community centre'). It must be noted that there was a significant improvement in a number of areas of Farouq's functioning before he achieved refugee status.

Another significant issue is the role of memory. A study was undertaken that aimed to investigate the consistency of autobiographical memory of people seeking asylum, to test the assumption that discrepancies in asylum seeker's accounts of persecution could mean that they are fabricating their stories. The results indicated that for participants with high levels of post-traumatic stress, the number of discrepancies increased with the length of time between interviews. In addition, accounts were more likely to be inconsistent in details that the individual considered as peripheral to their experience, rather than the details they considered central to the traumatic event: for example, dates, times, and other details are less likely to be remembered than say the details surrounding their detention, torture, or rape (Herlihy, Scragg and Turner, 2002). Therefore, inconsistent recall does not necessarily imply that individuals are fabricating their accounts of torture or other traumatic experience.

The patient's legal status also makes a difference to treatment outcomes because of the uncertainty surrounding status and fears of return for those still awaiting asylum decisions. This inevitably affects therapeutic progress because the individual is focused on realistic fears for the future and, therefore, is often unable to focus on the 'here and now'. Furthermore, the therapeutic interventions, such a CBT and other approaches, would be inadvisable where the patient is homeless or destitute (which can often be the case, depending on the current asylum laws). In such cases, therapeutic engagement needs to be more focused on creating and fostering a safe environment and the provision of practical support.

One of the most significant therapeutic developments in recent years of working with the aftermath of trauma across cultures has been the use of Narrative Exposure Therapy (NET) (see Schauer, Neuner, and Elbert 2011). NET has been developed and refined over the past decade as an integration of CBT and testimony therapy (TT), a short-term psychological treatment method that was especially developed for survivors of torture and other severe human rights violations. TT aims at the construction of a detailed and coherent report of the survivor's biography, including an explicit description of the traumatic events. The written testimony created by the survivor, in co-operation with a therapist, is used for documentary and political purposes in support of the survivor. The procedures of CBT and TT share many common features. As in CBT, prolonged exposure to the traumatic material is realized through reporting about it. This promotes the habituation of emotional and physiological reactions to reminders of the traumatic events and so reduces symptoms. But the focus of TT is not on the patient overcoming fears related to their experiences, but on the reconstruction of the shattered autobiographical memories of the traumatic experiences. NET is, therefore, a combination of these two approaches, and it has been used successfully in many cross-cultural settings, again by working closely with and training local professionals (e.g. social workers and teachers as lay therapists). It has also been developed for children (KIDNET) and again used in the wake of recent disasters and in refugee camps (see Appendix 2 for website details). Furthermore, the effectiveness of NET as a trauma therapy has been supported by a growing body of research.

Working with interpreters—some guidelines for mental health workers

◆ When booking the interpreter, try to provide as much information as possible to help the interpreting service to ensure they send an appropriate interpreter. For example, it is important not just to match the language but also to consider gender and ethnic affiliations. It is important for health workers to have a good working alliance with the interpreter, as well as with the patient.

◆ Check that the interpreter is acceptable to the patient—an obvious example where this might not be the case would be a male interpreter working with a female patient who has been raped. Also, interpreters sometimes speak the same language, but belong to a hostile ethnic group.

◆ Since interpreters may well know a great deal more than the therapist does about the patient's culture and background, they can also be an invaluable source of information about how the patient is likely to respond to particular questions or lines of enquiry.

◆ Patients tend to look at the therapist when he or she is speaking, but look at the interpreter when they themselves are speaking. This reduces the sense of having a direct conversation with the patient, and it underlines the fact that the interpreter is a third person in the session, whose sensitivity and responsiveness will have an impact on your work.

◆ Allow enough time for the interview because working with an interpreter takes longer: usually, allow 1½–2 hours for a session.

◆ Before commencing the appointment, it is important that the therapist explain the particular treatment model and how it works and informs the interpreter about the style of interpretation required.

◆ Topics covered in the interview are often distressing. Where possible, before the interview, the interpreter should be provided with background information about the patient, including the subject matter likely to be covered. A preinterview briefing will also give the interpreter the opportunity to brief you on possible cultural issues that might arise in the context of the discussion and any issues he or she may have in relation to the content to be discussed.

◆ Before the start of the appointment, consider seating arrangements so everyone can be properly and appropriately involved in the interview. This is particularly an issue for family appointments or appointments where there are likely to be several people in the room.

◆ If you have any concerns about an interpreter (e.g. the language or cultural match between the interpreter and patient, or you feel there may be tension between the interpreter and patient), it is helpful to let the interpreting service know this. This will help the service to find a more appropriate interpreter for the patient in the future, and it supports the service's quality monitoring.

◆ Ensure that the interpreter is aware of confidentiality, and has explained to the patient that he or she will treat everything discussed in the interview as strictly confidential.

◆ During the interview, use straightforward language, avoiding complex terminology or jargon.

◆ Make time available at the end of the session to discuss the case and the interpreter's feelings during the session. This can be brief, and it will allow the interpreter to give the therapist any additional perspectives he or she may have on the therapeutic encounter (e.g. the interpreter may have noticed that the patient was inhibited from speaking about something, perhaps in line with cultural norms). The 'debrief' should also help the interpreter mentally to 'exit' the appointment and relationship with the patient. The interpreter may need support to set boundaries so that they can exit their relationship with the patient at the end of the appointment (e.g. making sure the interpreter does not have to leave the building with the patient).

Working with asylum seekers and refugees—some guidelines for interpreters

◆ Therapy sessions are different from psychiatric assessment sessions. An important part of the work with people who have experienced traumatic events often includes the disclosure of shameful feelings and thoughts. This can only be done when trust has been established. This makes it important for them to have the same interpreter, wherever possible, over a course of treatment. It is important to let the therapist know as far in advance as possible about times when you will not be available, such as absences owing to other work commitments, holidays, and so on.

◆ As with all health-interpreting appointments, everything discussed in the sessions is confidential. It is important that patients are aware of this and feel confident that you will treat everything as confidential.

◆ Most therapists prefer interpreters, where possible, to use the 'first person' when translating the patient's words. You may like to check this with the therapist before you start the appointment; sometimes it is acceptable to convey the patient's story in the third person.

♦ It is important to translate everything the patient says, even if it seems irrelevant to what is being discussed at the time, but share any observations you may have about that experience.

♦ As an interpreter, you probably know much more than the therapist does about the patient's culture and cultural ways of thinking. This knowledge may be very important for the therapist to know. For example, it may help him or her to understand why the patient engages or responds to treatment in a certain way. If you have additional information that you think would be helpful for the therapist to know, please let them know. However, when doing so, it is important to be clear about when you are interpreting what the patient has said and when you are offering your own opinion.

♦ As with all interpreting assignments, you should not start discussions with the patient or give direct advice without first discussing it with the therapist in the first instance. The patient has to make decisions for him or herself.

♦ Often the phrasing of questions is extremely important, so you should translate as directly as possible, without adding, subtracting, or putting questions into another form.

♦ Try not to make open questions into leading questions (i.e. questions that require a yes/no answer). For example, an open question is 'How are you feeling'?; a leading question would be 'Are you feeling OK'?

♦ Silence during the sessions may be meaningful. Try not to repeat questions or 'push' the patient unless the therapist asks you to do so.

♦ If the patient asks you not to tell the therapist something, please tell the therapist that they have said this, before the patient has told you what it is they want you not to interpret.

♦ It is understandable and common for the patient to become upset. The therapist and interpreter should simply acknowledge and validate these feelings. Therefore, when the patient is upset, try to resist the urge to comfort the patient directly through touch or by saying, for example, 'it will be OK, don't cry'.

♦ Therapists are aware that it is not always possible to provide an exact word-for-word translation. Please explain to the therapist why a particular question is hard to ask in a language and suggest possible alternatives that are more appropriate.

♦ If you have any concerns about the patient, please tell the therapist.

♦ If you have questions or do not understand what the therapist is doing or why he or she is asking certain questions, then please ask the therapist at the end of the session when the patient has left. It is important that you have an understanding of what is happening.

◆ It is important to be aware that the work often involves discussing and describing highly disturbing and distressing situations, and that this may well have an emotional effect on you. Try to find ways of taking care of yourself emotionally when doing this work. In addition to this, the therapist should make time available at the end of the session to discuss the case and your own feelings during the session; this kind of debriefing can help you to manage difficult feelings about the session when you leave. Please ask your therapist to help you if you are experiencing any particular difficulties as a result of the work you have been doing.

Trauma and culture—the work of humanitarian aid agencies

The past decade has seen an increasing focus and consensus on the importance of providing what has become known as 'psychosocial support', following disasters and complex emergencies. Many non-governmental organizations (NGOs) have been actively involved in the delivery of psychosocial support programmes (PSPs, sometimes also referred to as psychological support programmes) in varied contexts and settings, whether it is following natural disasters, as in the case of the recent Tsunami, or in the wake of armed conflict. The term *psychosocial* has become the preferred term when describing interventions designed to impact positively on the mental health needs of those individuals and communities affected by complex emergencies, and, therefore, it will be used throughout the chapter. In addition, the field of psychosocial interventions is relatively young, and inevitably, there have been calls to determine the evidence base for such interventions. There have also been critiques of the notion of PSP, as there is a view that many communities affected by complex emergencies are resilient and thus have an innate capacity to heal themselves without external intervention. Inevitably, there have also been critiques of the appropriateness and what has often been perceived as the 'medicalized' nature of such interventions.

It is important to understand that individuals, communities, and societies not only cope with but also have the innate ability to adapt to adversity and to focus psychosocial interventions at building on these strengths. In 1991, the International Federation of Red Cross and Red Crescent Societies (IFRC) launched the Psychological Support Programme (PSP) as a crosscutting programme under the Health and Care Division. To assist the IFRC with the implementation of the programme, the Danish Red Cross and IFRC established the Reference Centre for Psychological Support as a centre of excellence in 1993. In November 2004, the centre changed its name to the

Reference Centre (RC) for Psychosocial Support, which has the following guiding principles:

◆ Assisting local initiatives, which will lead to a durable and meaningful change in the psychological well-being of people affected by disasters and stressful life events;

◆ Collaborating with Red Cross/Red Crescent National Societies to build sustainable psychosocial support programmes that are based on genuine local ownership, avoiding the creation of aid-dependent parallel structures;

◆ Working on the basis of locally identified needs, rather than on the reflexes of the aid community;

◆ Paying special attention to women and children, who are often the most vulnerable groups in a post-conflict situation, as well as to families with missing members; and

◆ Any discussion on the relationship between humanitarian aid providers and recipients should be based on the concept of respect for the prevailing culture and its mental health or psychosocial healing practices (IFRC Reference Centre for Psychosocial Support 2006).

Psychosocial interventions and enhancing resilience in complex emergencies

In complex emergencies, such as major disasters, especially those involving severe injuries, bereavement and loss, there will indeed be mental health consequences for many survivors. This would be especially so where the social infrastructure has been compromised. Whatever mental health systems existed before the emergency may now be insufficient to meet the multifaceted needs of communities affected. Mollica and colleagues (2004), only a few days before the Asian tsunami of 2004, urged countries throughout the world to prepare themselves to deal with 'Mental health in complex emergencies'. It is noteworthy that the authors were not calling for armies of counsellors to be drafted in or for Western models of therapy to be utilized, but acknowledging the impact that disasters can have on individuals, families, and communities.

The concept of PSP has become firmly established in the repertoire of humanitarian organizations' interventions following complex emergencies. There is an expectation that individuals and communities following catastrophe are resilient, but there is also an understanding borne out by a considerable body of evidence that there are mental health consequences for some survivors. The loss of life and forced migration suffered by many communities following the Asian tsunami, focused national and international agencies on the need to provide appropriate psychosocial care from the very beginning. The early arguments and criticisms surrounding PSP and early interventions paled into insignificance when faced by the urgent need to reduce distress and prevent the development of longer term mental health problems. In the wake of the death, destruction, multiple bereavements, and losses, including homes and livelihoods, doing nothing was not an option. Lessons had also been learned following the mental health response after the earthquake that devastated the city of Barn in Southern Iran, destroying 85% of the city. An estimated 26,000 people were killed, and a further 30,000 were injured. This response was delivered early and was the product of much planning and preparation for just such a disaster. Knowing that the region was vulnerable to earthquakes, the Department of Mental Health in the Ministry of Health in Iran, in collaboration with the Iranian Red Crescent, started conducting a series of workshops for relief workers in the basic skills of psychosocial support. Further training was also facilitated by UNICEF and the Centre for Crisis Psychology in Norway (Yule 2006).

This example is of course one of many illustrating that PSPs do not focus on PTSD and are not restricted to a conventional Eurocentric view of suffering and distress. All PSPs are designed in collaboration with local agencies and communities, especially those conducted through the International Red Cross and Red Crescent Societies' Reference Centre for Psychosocial Support. A key element is, and always has been, the facilitation and enhancement of local resources and communities, together with capacity building. Requests for PSPs come from a wide variety of Red Cross and Red Crescent National Societies; a recent example has been within the Somali Red Crescent, which has been developing a culturally sensitive framework for the development and delivery of psychosocial training for its volunteers. In many developing countries, the local Red Cross/Red Crescent Society often provides basic health and social care, something in the West that is often taken for granted.

Some have argued that the transfer of Western concepts and techniques (e.g. to war-affected societies) risks perpetuating the colonial status of non-Western mind-sets, as every culture has its own frameworks for mental health and norms for help seeking at times of crisis. This argument is based on making distinctions between Western 'Eurocentric' cultures and cultures in non-industrialized countries, and while it may appear a straightforward distinction, it is far from being the case. Many societies have chosen to adapt mental health concepts developed by Western psychology and prefer corresponding intervention methods, often in combination with traditional healing, as has been seen in South Africa. Similarly, in many rural areas in European countries, traditional healing techniques for physical and mental complaints have remained popular.

There is evidence that in some instances whereby an integrated model of intervention using the framework described above has had significant utility.

As referred to earlier, following the earthquake of 2003, in Bam, Iran, the Children and War Recovery Manual (see Appendix 2 for website details) was adapted with local collaboration and used by the psychosocial teams, based on previous experiences and training. This formed the basis for trauma counselling interventions based on cognitive behavioural exercises and included brief group exercises over four sessions with about 960 children and 742 adults. About 1500 local mental health professionals and teachers were trained to provide brief interventions. The evaluations, postintervention questionnaires, and clinician reports indicated that 85% (some 55,000) of the survivors benefited from the sessions (Yule 2006). Many interventions utilize psychoeducational strategies, such as information about the psychological impact of traumatic events and related supportive advice. Support and guidance are likely to cover reassurance about immediate distress, information about the likely course of symptoms, strategies for effective coping, health, and psychosocial support in emergency settings. The aim is to systemize the field by development of coherent practice-based guidance. This work is currently being done by the Inter-Agency Standing Committee (IASC) task force on Mental Health and Psychosocial Support in Emergency settings (2007). The IASC is a unique interagency forum for coordination, policy development, and decision making involving the key UN and non-UN humanitarian partners. The IASC was established in June 1992 in response to a United Nations General Assembly Resolution on the strengthening of humanitarian assistance. The General Assembly Resolution affirmed its role as the primary mechanism for interagency coordination of humanitarian assistance. Under the leadership of the IASC, the United Nations develops humanitarian policies, agrees on a clear division of responsibility for the various aspects of humanitarian assistance, identifies and addresses gaps in response, and advocates for effective application of humanitarian principles. Together with the Executive Committee for Humanitarian Affairs (ECHA), the IASC forms the key strategic coordination mechanism among major humanitarian agencies.

Psychosocial support following disasters: a case study

On 8 October 2005, a powerful earthquake measuring 7.6 on the Richter scale hit Northern Pakistan and Northern India; the tremors were felt across the region from Kabul in Afghanistan to Delhi. In less than a minute, whole towns and villages were reduced to rubble, and landslides had washed away roads and villages on mountainsides. The death toll was more than 80,000, with over 4 million people made homeless. The European Commission Humanitarian Office (ECHO) funded a psychosocial programme following the disaster, as the government of Pakistan and all relevant stakeholders involved in the relief operation recognized the urgency of addressing not only the physical and material needs of those affected but also the emotional and psychosocial needs of the population. The funding allowed the Danish Red Cross (DRC) and the Pakistan Red Crescent Society (PRCS), supported by the IFRC to initiate a psychosocial programme in four refugee camps in the North-West frontier and in Islamabad in November 2005. The initial assessment, carried out immediately after the earthquake, found the disaster had also caused enormous psychological distress because of significant loss of life, shelter, and livelihood, not to mention multiple losses in many cases.

The immediate priority following the earthquake was to provide food, shelter, and medical aid to all those affected. The majority of the population in the area affected by the earthquake lived in remote and scattered villages with a limited and basic infrastructure in terms of communication, transport, and other services. The small and isolated communities affected, sustained a living through the land, often eking out a basic and simple existence. The literacy rate in the most affected areas was low, with women leading secluded lives, often rarely interacting with the outside world other than their extended family. In addition, some of the affected areas had been isolated as a result of the long-lasting conflict between India and Pakistan in Kashmir. The harsh winter conditions hampered immediate reconstruction and prevented the population from regaining their livelihoods and other day-to-day activities. A large part of the affected population also had to spend the winter months in temporary camps away from their place of origin.

The psychosocial team's assessment indicated that many were experiencing what would be considered normal responses to a disaster of such proportion. Many felt disbelief at what had happened, finding it difficult to absorb the enormity of the situation and to assess the damage and loss for themselves, their families, and communities. Initially the emphasis was on practical issues, such as recovering the remains of loved ones, arranging burial ceremonies, and other cultural rituals. In this remote area of Pakistan, religion plays an important part in the traditional lifestyle of these isolated communities.

At assessment, the psychosocial team was able to establish many of the challenges presented when organizing a PSP to facilitate culturally appropriate coping strategies. It was decided at an early stage that it was of great importance to involve individuals, families, and communities within the camp in the decisions regarding psychosocial initiatives, so that they could express what they regarded as helpful in the facilitation of a healing process, and to enhance their natural resilience. The team was also very aware of the significance of religion and the role of women in a very traditional and rural setting of Pakistan.

The programme began in November 2005, and it was implemented within the biggest refugee camps, utilizing 16 PRCS field workers, a programme manager, and a field team coordinator. All these individuals were recruited and trained using context-specific psychosocial models and were working in collaboration with local NGOs who agreed to provide training, professional supervision, and support to field workers during the project period. Within 3 months, four teams had generated awareness about the psychological reactions to trauma, established a variety of social activities, and organized volunteers in four of the large camps. The volunteers were initially supported until they felt able to work independently, before other similar activities were established in surrounding villages and communities. Activities were all based on participatory assessments and knowledge gained from focused interviews and multiple meetings with the target communities. The most common activity was the psychoeducational sessions for different groups (e.g. children of different ages, women, and men). Social activities were also initiated, aimed at creating a safe and culturally appropriate environment, where different groups could meet, share problems and concerns, and be actively involved in the recovery and rehabilitation process.

The PRCS had not previously been involved in psychosocial activities and subsequently did not have any staff members trained in this area, or any who could be transferred to the new programme. In the event, all field workers were new employees having been newly introduced to the PRCS and the Red Crescent movement, receiving intensive training in required knowledge and skills. The psychosocial team found that experience and lessons learned from other PSPs meant it was important to create specific modules designed for each of the project areas. For example, women in the affected areas, not being used to attending groups where they shared feelings and feedback, were in groups facilitated by women. Widows and orphans were often absorbed into extended families and not seen as particularly vulnerable. However, the new dynamic created by social, emotional, and economic situations in a new family can be extremely problematic and result in violence and abuse. Therefore, this was a significant challenge and was addressed by using field workers and volunteers drawn from the local communities. At the time of writing, the projects continue, and there are plans to develop further expertise for staff, to strengthen the PRCS and engage in capacity building, ultimately incorporating psychosocial support and activities within the PRCS Heath Department.

Conclusions

As can be seen, the concept of trauma across cultures is a complex subject for a variety of reasons, but there is an acknowledgement of the human condition. The impact of traumatic events on individuals, families, and communities seems well understood by people from non-Western cultural backgrounds, even in the face of variations in concepts of health and healing. There is reason to believe that reactions to traumatic events do have a degree of universality. The International Federation of Red Cross and Red Crescent Society's Reference Centre for Psycho-social Support has been responding to requests from different countries to establish psychosocial programmes to complement other activities, such as community-based first-aid. Across cultures, human beings have similar reactions to distressing, stressful, and traumatic events, but their responses may differ—as may interventions.

References

Frontex. (2015). *Annual risk analysis 2015*. http://frontex.europa.eu/assets/Publications/Risk_Analysis/Annual_Risk_Analysis_2015.pdf[Accessed 31 March 2016].

Herlihy, J., Scragg, P., and Turner, S. (2002). Discrepancies in autobiographical memories—implications for the assessment of asylum seekers: repeated interviews study. *British Medical Journal* **324**, 324–327.

Inter-Agency Standing Committee. (2007). *IASC guidelines on mental health and psychosocial support in emergency settings*. Geneva: IASC.

IFRC. (2015). *Remembering the 2005 Pakistan earthquake*. http://www.ifrc.org/en/news-and-media/news-stories/asia-pacific/pakistan/remembering-the-2005-pakistan-earthquake-69487/ [Accessed 31 May 2016].

McCall, G. J. and Resick, P. A. (2003). A pilot study of PTSD symptoms among Kalahari bushmen. *Journal of Traumatic Stress* **16**(5), 445–450.

Mollica, R. R., Lopez Cardoza, B., Osofsky, H. J., Raphael, B., Ager, A., and Salama, P. (2004). Mental health in complex emergencies. *Lancet* **364**, 2058–2067.

O'Reilly, D., and Stevenson, M. (2003). Mental health in Northern Ireland: have 'the Troubles' made it worse? *Journal of Epidemiology and Community Health* **57**(7), 488.

Reference Centre for Psychosocial Support. (2006). *Guiding principles*. (http://psp.drk.dk/sw26837.asp) [Accessed 8 September 2016].

Regel, S., and Berliner, P. (2007). Current perspectives on assessment and therapy with survivors of torture: the use of a cognitive behavioural approach. *European Journal of Psychotherapy and Counselling* **9**(3), 289–299.

Schauer, M., Neuner, F., and Elbert, T. (2011). *Narrative exposure therapy: a short-term intervention for traumatic stress disorders after war, terror or torture*. Washington, DC: Hogrefe & Huber.

Stroebe, M. S. (1992). Coping with bereavement: a review of the grief work hypothesis. *Omega: Journal of Death and Dying* **26**, 19–42.

Terheggen, M. A, Stroebe M. S., and Kleber R. J. (2001). Western conceptualisations and Eastern experience: a cross-cultural study of traumatic stress reactions among Tibetan refugees in India. *Journal of Traumatic Stress* **14**(2), 391–403.

UNHCHR. (1984). *Inhuman or degrading treatment or punishment*. http://www.ohchr.org/EN/ProfessionalInterest/Pages/CAT.aspx [Accessed 8 September 2016].

UNHCR. (2016a). The sea route to Europe: the Mediterranean passage in the age of refugees. http://www.unhcr.org/5592bd059.html [Accessed 1 March 2016].

UNHCR. (2016b). World at war: Global trends, forced displacement in 2014. http://www.unhcr.org/556725e69.html [Accessed1 March 2016].

UNHCR. (2016c). Figures at a glance. Retrieved from http://www.unhcr.org/figures-at-a-glance.html [Accessed1 March 2016].

United Nations. (1948). Universal declaration of human rights. http://www.un.org/en/documents/udhr/ [Accessed1 March 2016].

World Health Organization. (1986). *The health hazards of organized violence. Report on a WHO Meeting*. Veldhoven. 22–25 April 1986.

World Health Organization. (1992). *The ICD-10 classification of mental and behavioural disorders: clinical descriptions and diagnostic guidelines*. Geneva: WHO.

World Health Organization. (1997). Considering conflict. Concept paper for first Health as a Bridge for Peace, Consultative Meeting. www.who.int/hac/techguidance/hbp/considering_conflict/en/ [Accessed 24 April 2007].

Wilson, J. P., and Drozdek, B., eds. (2004). *Broken spirits: the treatment of traumatized asylum seekers, refugees, war and torture victims.* New York: Brunner-Routledge.

Yule, W. (2006). Theory, training and timing: psychosocial interventions in complex emergencies. *International Review of Psychiatry 18*(3), 259–264.

Helping survivors and their families

8

Early intervention strategies

Mental health promotion

> ## ➲ Key Points
>
> - Immediately following trauma and adversity, and in the hours subsequently, people are often in a state of shock and disbelief and are confused and disoriented.
> - Over the following days and weeks, people may continue to be confused and disoriented. At this point social support from others is important.
> - Timing of help is very important. At some points, people need information; at other points, emotional support; and at other points, practical support.
> - In the early stages, information, advice, reassurance, and guidance about common reactions, the course of these reactions, and signposting for further help are what individuals and families often find most helpful.
> - Conventional counselling or therapy within the first 6–8 weeks of exposure to a traumatic event is often not indicated or helpful, but professional advice and help should be sought if common reactions do not subside in intensity, frequency, or duration.
> - A variety of strategies can be adopted in order to attempt to mitigate against further adverse reactions or complications from developing.
> - Many organizations (e.g. the emergency services and the military) use peers to support and assist personnel exposed to extremely stressful incidents.

Helping in the aftermath

There has been an ongoing debate over the past 2 decades as to how best to help people in the aftermath of trauma and adversity. As we have seen in the earlier chapters, not everyone exposed to a traumatic experience will go on to develop severe and long-lasting problems, but others will. We know that one of the most important differences between people who develop problems and those who don't is social support; so it seems sensible to try to offer support to people.

There is a strong human desire to assist victims of a trauma and attempt to try to undo or ease their pain and suffering. Many academics, psychologists, psychiatrists, and psychotherapists would probably agree that prevention of future problems might not always be possible, but there are strategies and supportive interventions, when used appropriately, which may help individuals (and families) at an early stage. In this chapter, we will look at what individuals, families, and organizations can do to assist those affected.

We will look at what individuals and families may find helpful, especially following a sudden traumatic bereavement following a road-traffic collision, homicide, natural or human-made disaster. We will also look at what organizations, such as the emergency services, offer employees exposed to trauma in the workplace. Finally, some ideas, thoughts, and observations on helpful strategies at an early stage will be outlined.

A brief history of early interventions for trauma

The basic framework was drawn from 'crisis-intervention' theories. The period immediately following exposure to a trauma may be considered to constitute a crisis. A crisis can be seen as a state of temporary destabilization and sometimes breakdown in an individual's ability to cope with usual needs and, as mentioned earlier, problem solving is affected, as may the ability to process and make sense of new information. So a crisis can be caused by an experience of threat, loss, or factors that overwhelm or threaten to overwhelm usual coping responses.

A significant influencing factor was work developed by Lindemann following support offered to victims of the Coconut Grove Nightclub Fire in Boston, Massachusetts, in 1944, where over 400 people lost their lives. This work was further developed and broadened by Caplan (1961) to be utilized in more widely defined potentially stressful or traumatic events.

Sadly, many individuals and families affected by traumatic experiences, unfortunately tend not to access help and support until much later and when problems have become entrenched. However, in the event of a major disaster, help and support tends to be offered relatively soon. For example, many major cities and counties in the UK will have Crisis Support teams to address the practical, social, and emotional needs of those affected. This is also the aim of the British Red Cross Psychosocial Support team established in 2004. We would recommend that individuals and families affected by traumatic events such as those described throughout this book seek assistance and support at the earliest available opportunity to avoid complications in the longer term. Whilst we appreciate that many individuals are resilient and can mobilize their own support, we also recognize that many cannot or are unable to do this for a variety of reasons. Our extensive experience of seeing people in the relatively early stages post exposure to trauma indicate that education, information, and structured social support such as that indicated and described after traumatic bereavement (see Chapter 4) have the potential to mitigate against future adverse psychological reactions (Dyregrov and Regel, 2012).

Psychological debriefing and related peer support: a brief historical overview

Many organizations, such as the emergency services, banks following armed robbery, and the military, use methods of early intervention for their personnel. The methods were developed over 20 years ago, but are often slightly modified and tailored to meet individual organizational needs.

In the 1980s, the idea of helping people in crisis in occupational settings was taken a stage further and developed by Jeffrey Mitchell as a peer support intervention for emergency service personnel in the USA. The framework became known (and still is) as Critical Incident Stress Management (CISM): it was further developed and refined over the past 2 decades and since been clearly described as a 'comprehensive, systematic and integrated multi-component crisis-intervention package that enables individuals and groups to receive assessment of need, practical support and follow-up following exposure to traumatic events in the workplace. In addition, it facilitates the early detection and treatment of post traumatic and other psychological reactions'.

CISM in its current form was originally designed to provide peer support, education, and monitoring of individuals and groups of emergency workers, such as fire fighters and police officers, exposed to potentially traumatic experiences through the course of their work (Everley and Mitchell 2003, 2008). Emergency service workers may present differently from other trauma survivors in whom a single traumatic event is the primary focus of their reactions. The armed forces are also more commonly involved in peacekeeping or humanitarian duties and, as a result, they can be exposed to considerable human suffering, with no immediate threat to themselves, and, in this respect, are increasingly similar to emergency workers. Typical risk scenarios in emergency workers include:

◆ Repeated experience of a variety of traumatic incidents that entail varying degrees of a sense of personal threat, often combined with the witnessing of harm or death to others, rather than experience of a single incident.

◆ An incident where the individual makes some personal identification with a victim or event.

◆ Incidents that are sudden and catastrophic and give little time for mental mobilization or preparedness (e.g. finding that the scene or event they are attending overwhelms their emotional and physical resources).

◆ Contextual life events—one or more personal stressors occurring around the time of the work-related incident that preoccupy the individual (e.g. recent loss and bereavement, family ill health, or relationship or financial problems). These will have an impact upon the resilience and coping strategies of the individual.

◆ Repeated intense exposures over a period leading to accumulated risk.

◆ Major terrorist incidents and disasters with multiple loss of life, especially those including children.

◆ Combat experience.

CISM programmes within these organizations comprise a number of elements, which include:

◆ Precrisis education—for individuals and groups within organizations.

◆ Assessment—of the nature, potential, and actual impact of the incident on individuals and groups involved.

◆ Defusing—a brief peer-group support meeting within the first 24 hours or at the end of a shift.

◆ Critical Incident Stress Debriefing (CISD)—a structured group meeting held 72 hours to 14 days post incident.

◆ Specialist follow-up for ongoing psychological therapy support, if necessary—usually provided 'in-house' by organizations or out-sourced where necessary.

Controversy arose because attention was focused upon the CISD component of CISM. CISD is a structured form of crisis intervention that involves a discussion and review of the traumatic event or critical incident, followed by information, advice, and guidance on common reactions to trauma, as well as the course of these reactions and signposting as to where further support will be available, should that be necessary.

The term *psychological debriefing* (PD) was coined in 1989 by Atle Dyregrov, the director of the Centre of Crisis Psychology, Norway, and one of the founder members of the European Society of Traumatic Stress Studies who had developed a similar technique. Dyregrov (1989) defined PD as '. . . *a group meeting arranged for the purpose of integrating profound personal experiences both on the cognitive, emotional and group level, and thus preventing the development of adverse reactions*'.

Since then the terms *CISM* and *PD* (especially in Europe) have become interchangeable. The main difference (apart from the names of some of the later phases) is that Dyregrov places more emphasis on the process of the meeting than does Mitchell. The latter has also been developed within a European context and, therefore, it reflects a different tradition for groups and structure than those in the USA. The other difference is the use of the word *psychological*, which, in some organizational and cultural contexts, may have negative connotations. This became the focus of attention for research because it was erroneously perceived that this particular aspect of CISM would (a) alleviate the symptoms of post-traumatic stress disorder (PTSD) per se and (b) it was a 'stand-alone' process. For the purposes of this chapter and for the sake of clarity, the term *PD* will be used rather than *CISD* because it has been widely described as such in the literature and was used as the working title of the British Psychological Society's Report on Psychological Debriefing.

The most common technique of PD is a structured meeting, facilitated through a series of seven phases of PD:

◆ Introduction.

◆ Facts.

◆ Thoughts.

◆ Reactions.

◆ Normalization.

◆ Future planning and coping.

◆ Disengagement.

PD typically takes 1.5–3.0 hours to facilitate and is usually held 72 hours to 14 days post incident. The aim of PD is to:

◆ Provide education about common reactions to traumatic events and the course of these reactions.

◆ Assist individuals to begin the process of coming to terms with the incident/event.

◆ Indicate resources for further help and support, if and where necessary, and facilitate early help seeking, if appropriate.

◆ Provide social support and promote recovery; enhance natural resilience and personal growth.

PD was never intended as a 'stand-alone' intervention or as a substitute for counselling or psychotherapy. It is also often suggested that PD is of little benefit or a 'suitable treatment' for those suffering from PTSD, which is of course true. The reason why PD would be of little benefit is that it was never intended to be used with PTSD sufferers. It was intended as an educative crisis-intervention strategy, to be used for emergency services personnel (e.g. fire fighters, paramedics, police officers, and similar occupational groups), within the first 2–4 weeks following their exposure to an incident that would have been assessed to have the potential to impact their mental health and well-being. As we have seen earlier, PTSD can only be diagnosed 1 month after exposure to the traumatic event.

You will see that these methods of debriefing are about providing people with information, guidance, and advice as to what to expect. Certainly, for some people, at certain points, this is extremely valuable to do. But, PD is not a form of therapy for the treatment of post-traumatic stress. Sometimes, the media has created confusion by labelling it as 'counselling'.

Current use of CISM and PD within organizations

Current evidence at the time of writing suggests that many organizations, especially the emergency services and some sections of the military in the UK and abroad, continue to utilize CISM and PD as part of their post-incident support measures for personnel. Around the late-1980s, London's Metropolitan Police and many other police forces in the UK utilized PD, but adapted the technique from Mitchell and Dyregrov, which became known as the three-stage model. It is comprised of:

◆ Facts (equating to the Introduction and Facts phase of PD).

◆ Feelings (equating to the Thoughts and Reactions phase of PD).

◆ Future (equating to the Normalization, Future Planning/Coping, and Disengagement phases of PD).

Whilst this adaptation of the technique was in use for a number of years, the current focus is to retrain many peer support teams in CISM/PD using Dyregrov's approach. In view of the past controversy and the NICE guidelines, there has also been a trend for some organizations to develop new CISM models. As a result, CISM continues to be used by a number of organizations, but it is referred to in a variety of different ways. Below are a number of relatively new examples that describe early interventions very similar to CISM processes with some adaptations. For example:

- **Trauma Risk Management (TRiM)**—developed by two mental health professionals for the British Royal Marines, it is described as a post-traumatic management strategy, based upon peer-group assessment for hierarchical organizations. It also contains all the CISM components and utilizes aspects of the three-stage technique of PD developed in the late 1980s. This form of CISM has been adopted by some organizations in the UK.

- **Battlemind Debriefing**—an intervention (and training) developed by the US military, adapted from and based on Mitchell's CISD technique. Their research demonstrated that brief early interventions post deployment have the potential to be effective with at-risk occupational groups.

- **Psychological First Aid (PFA)**—has been defined as the use of pragmatic interventions delivered in the first 4 weeks to individuals experiencing acute stress reactions or those at risk of being unable to regain their functional equilibrium. It is meant to be embedded in systemic public health and emergency response systems. The origins of PFA are drawn from models of crisis intervention as described previously. The primary objectives of PFA include establishing safety, reducing acute stress reactions, aiding adaptive coping, and facilitating problem-solving processes and signposts for survivors to other resources needed. It has been recommended for aid workers and in disaster mental health settings. Thus, there are many similarities to CISM.

- **Emotional Decompression**—a relatively recent but little used addition, it is also is a hybrid of the three-stage technique and seven-stage PD technique.

Therefore, on closer inspection, models that purport to be offering different solutions to post-trauma support in the workplace are all practising CISM and PD under new acronyms. It also means that many organizations are offering similar post-incident support systems but modifying the process to suit their organizational context and needs, such as TRiM, which is well suited to a military context. Most recently, the term *peer support* has been used to describe a variety of interventions and methods of supporting personnel in high-risk professions. The Australian Centre for Post Traumatic Mental Health developed guidelines for peer support in the workplace in 2011. These guidelines can be used to develop peer support programmes and highlight areas for further research.

The research and current recommendations

Only two studies have suggested that CISM/ PD may not be helpful, and they have promoted the idea that the approach has the potential to cause harm. These studies, however, were conducted with hospitalized individuals who had experienced a road-traffic collision or a burn trauma. They were not conducted with groups that the interventions were originally intended for, and have been the source of much debate and controversy in the field. It has also been recognized that the studies have methodological flaws; thus, further research is needed. It was also noted in the NICE guidelines, that none of the studies that showed negative effects contained any descriptions of the training given to those carrying out the interventions, as these involve a unique set of skills. The 2015 update of the NICE guidelines has clearly indicated that it may now be appropriate to reconsider recommendations, which state that debriefing should not be routine practice. There are nevertheless a number of studies that have also shown CISM/PD to be helpful and well accepted by those receiving the intervention, and that CISM/PD does not cause harm. Thus, when it is used in high-risk occupational settings, such as the emergency services, the aims are usually as follows:

♦ A practical means of providing social and organizational support.

♦ Helps contextualize the traumatic experience.

♦ Facilitates emotional processing (the 'repacking of the bag'—which we will discuss below).

♦ Helps challenge perception of guilt and self-blame, where present.

♦ Facilitates and encourages the use of appropriate coping strategies.

♦ Facilitates early help seeking—thus hopefully preventing possible psychological complications in the longer term.

♦ Helps to diminish the impact of the traumatic event.

The reasons for providing social support are based on overwhelming evidence from 30 years of research that it is a major protective factor following major life events or trauma. There are different types of social support: informational, practical, and emotional. The type of social support required depends on the context and individual needs, which will vary over time. It is important to match support provision to needs.

Wherever it is offered, it is not the aim or intention to prevent or reduce symptoms of PTSD, but as a means of providing social and organizational support. There are numerous other examples where early interventions are offered to provide practical, emotional, and social support following exposure to traumatic events. In these cases, what is offered will not be psychological debriefing, but often the general principles of support offered are the same. The most notable example was following the Tsunami of 2005. Since then, the British Red Cross has worked closely with the British Foreign and Commonwealth Office (FCO) to provide psychosocial support to UK nationals affected by incidents abroad. The British Red Cross Psychosocial Support Team (PST) consists of professionals drawn from a variety of settings, both within the British Red Cross and externally from organizations such as health and social care services in the UK with a health, mental health, and social care background. The British Red Cross PST has since responded to a significant number of international crises in the past 12 years to provide UK nationals with psychosocial support. These have included natural disasters and terrorist-related events. The aim of the PST is to provide practical, social, and emotional support in line with the NICE guidelines in the aftermath of a major life crisis. In addition, the use of early interventions and structured social support are also helpful with individuals and families following traumatic bereavement (as outlined in Chapter 4). Many Red Cross and Red Crescent national societies and the International Committee of the Red Cross (ICRC) provide similar forms of support at times of major crisis and disaster (Regel, Dyregrov, and Joseph 2007).

In summary, therefore, the fundamental guidelines for early support that should be followed when working with individuals and groups after exposure to traumatic events in the workplace offered by numerous organizations are:

◆ Early support should be based on good assessment.

◆ Provide pragmatic psychological support in an empathic manner, information about common reactions and course of these reactions, advice on coping strategies, and 'signposts' for further help.

◆ Individuals who show a continued increase in the frequency, intensity, and duration of any common or adverse reactions should be offered/may benefit from formal intervention.

◆ An approach that takes account of an individual's natural resilience.

◆ Attendance at support meetings should be voluntary.

Thus the majorities of peer support programmes and initiatives, whatever they are called, have the objective of providing social and organizational support, which has a strong evidence base as a protective factor following exposure to traumatic events.

The process of recovery

Just as there are many normal ways of reacting to traumatic experiences, so, too, there are many ways of dealing with the impact of these events. One way of understanding this is to consider the following analogy.

When individuals are exposed to or experience traumatic events, they often experience a range of thoughts and emotions that they are unable to deal with, or make sense of, at the time of the trauma, for various reasons: for example, they may be frightened, shocked, numb, in pain, worried about loved ones, being cut out of a car, or being interviewed by the police. As a result, these thoughts or emotions are often hurriedly 'packed' in an imaginary bag and taken away with them from the scene of the trauma. However, this 'emotional luggage', because it has been hurriedly and not well packed, may frequently burst open from time to time or when it is 'knocked against' something. This is often experienced as distressing thoughts, images, nightmares, and other emotions, which they have tried to push out of their mind because they find them so upsetting. Common examples would be when they are exposed to situations or events that resemble aspects of the trauma or the trauma itself.

What many people do over time is unpack and repack their bag, thereby helping themselves to come to terms with and make sense of their traumatic experience. Inevitably, there are things they have to keep (e.g. the traumatic experience). Eventually they will be able to dispense with many items (e.g. guilt and anger) and rearrange others; this might involve them having differ-ent perceptions of their experience. The aim is to be able, eventually, to carry the bag without it bursting open unexpectedly and be able to open it and view the contents at any time without undue distress. In addition, because this act of 'bursting open' is happening much less frequently, the bag becomes hardly noticeable. However, whilst the unpacking and repacking is a painful process, this becomes easier over time.

Ways of facilitating this process are through a variety of CISM and peer support interventions in occupational settings and through the many Red Cross initiatives described herein.

Conclusions

Being aware of the psychological trajectory of the response within the first 4–12 weeks is helpful because early reactions influence whether people go on to develop severe and chronic problems. If the initial distress is steadily diminishing in frequency, intensity, and duration, then it is likely that the person will recover well. However, problems early on, particularly to do with avoidance, can indicate the development of later complications.

Individuals and families affected by traumatic bereavement may benefit from structured social support as described earlier, but the time frame for the course of normal reactions is much longer, and recovery is influenced by a range of complex environmental and contextual factors (see Chapter 4). A mental health assessment may be appropriate to assess and determine indi-vidual needs, with attention being paid to risk assessment and other factors, such as previous and current vulnerabilities and the presence or otherwise of social support.

References

Australian Centre for Posttraumatic Mental Health. (2011). *Development of guidelines on peer support using the Delphi methodology.* (www.acpmh.unimelb.edu.au). [Accessed 9 September 2016].

Caplan, G. (1961). *An approach to community mental health.* New York: Grune and Stratton.

Dyregrov, A. (1989). Caring for helpers in disaster situations: psychological debriefing. *Disaster Management* 2(1), 25–30.

Dyregrov, A. and Regel, S. (2012). Early interventions following exposure to traumatic events-implications for practice from recent research. *Journal of Loss and Trauma: International Perspectives on Stress & Coping* 17(3), 271–2917.

Everley, G. S. and Mitchell, J. T. (2008). *Integrative crisis intervention and disaster mental health*. Ellicott City, MD: Chevron Publishing. (This book presents a general overview of Critical Incident Stress Management and Critical Incident Stress Debriefing, which is useful for the emergency services.)

Lindemann, E. (1944). Symptomatology and management of acute grief. *American Journal of Psychiatry* 101, 141–148.

Mitchell, J. T., and Everly, G. S. (2003). Critical incident stress management and critical incident stress debriefings: evolutions, effects and outcomes. In: Raphael, B., and Wilson, J. P., eds., *Psychological debriefing: theory, practice and evidence*. 2nd ed. Cambridge: Cambridge University Press. 71–90.

National Institute for Clinical Excellence (NICE). (2005). Post-traumatic stress disorder (PTSD): the management of PTSD in adults and children in primary and secondary care. London: Gaskell (www.nice.org.uk). [Accessed 9 September 2016].

Regel, S., and Dyregrov, A. (2012). Commonalities and new directions in post trauma support interventions: from pathology to the promotion of post traumatic growth. In: Hughes, R., Kinder, A., and Cooper, C., eds., *International handbook of workplace trauma support*. London: Wiley-Blackwell. 48–68

Regel, S., Dyregrov, A., and Joseph, S. (2007). Psychological debriefing in cross cultural contexts: ten implications for practice. *International Journal of Emergency Mental Health* 9(1):37–45.

9

Treatment for post-traumatic stress

➲ Key Points

- ◆ Post-traumatic stress disorder (PTSD) can be effectively treated with trauma-focused psychological interventions such as cognitive behavioural therapy (CBT).
- ◆ Medication should not usually be used as the first line of treatment for PTSD sufferers, but it may be helpful if (a) the person does not respond to psychological approaches and (b) lives under serious current threat of further trauma. Medications, especially anti-depressants, are often helpful as an adjunct to psychological treatment.
- ◆ Medication should not be used with children and adolescents to treat PTSD.
- ◆ Eye movement desensitization and reprocessing (EMDR) can be an effective treatment technique for treatment of PTSD.
- ◆ Other psychological treatment approaches may also be helpful to people who have experienced trauma, depending on individual needs.
- ◆ Existential and humanistic therapies can also help people to come to terms with changes in their lives.
- ◆ Litigation can often affect the course of psychological treatment.

Introduction

As we have seen, common post-traumatic stress reactions in some cases can develop into the chronic and disabling condition we have described in detail earlier as PTSD. Furthermore, there is a significant impact on not only individuals but also their partners, families, and relationships in general. Their ability to work, socialize, and lead active, productive lives and contribute to society, as they previously did, may be seriously affected, often for many years. In addition, secondary mental health problems, such as depression, anxiety, panic attacks, phobias, and alcohol and drug abuse, can also complicate the problem. Financial hardship, social isolation, and the breakdown or loss of support networks are all common occurrences. Physical injury (this was explored in more detail in Chapter 6) and personal losses can further complicate matters. Usually many sufferers present to their general practitioner (GP) months and sometimes years after the trauma. However, even when they seek help earlier, PTSD may go unrecognized. A research survey conducted after the 7/7 London Bombings suggested that PTSD may be under recognized in primary care settings (Brewin et al. 2008). This result was in keeping with a similar earlier study with 7/7 survivors and studies conducted in other countries, which have shown that PTSD is often under recognized in public mental health services. There may be a variety of reasons why this low recognition occurs, which may include the following:

◆ Time constraints and lack of information in GP surgeries.

◆ PTSD sufferers may be reluctant to inform their GP, as they often find talking about their experience extremely distressing.

◆ People suffering the effects of a traumatic experience may not be aware of the condition of PTSD.

◆ Sufferers often do not understand what is happening (as in Laura's story previously) but have developed unhelpful coping strategies, such as avoidance of reminders of the event, and this may include not seeking help for fear of having to discuss their experiences.

◆ Press and media coverage often represents the impact of traumatic experiences on individuals in a simplistic way, misrepresenting or confusing facts about the condition or the interventions used, often suggesting that help seeking is a sign of weakness, as characterized by the article headline in one major Sunday newspaper, which read, 'A stiff upper lip beats stress counselling'.

◆ Many feel they have to overcome their problems on their own.

◆ Many feel ashamed over the event and their responses.

◆ Children and adolescents may hide symptoms from parents.

◆ Many are not aware that help is available for psychological responses to trauma and that PTSD is a treatable condition.

Of course, the longer the condition continues the more chronic and intense the symptoms become. The mental and behavioural avoidance becomes more entrenched and sleep becomes more disturbed, often with disturbing dreams, and irritability, concentration, and physical symptoms become more marked. Relationship difficulties deepen, and other emotional states, such as anger, guilt, sadness, and emotional numbing, are ever present. Sometimes the more chronic and disabling the symptoms, the more difficult the road to recovery can be. However, it must be emphasized that this should not put anyone off from seeking help, as the length of time between the trauma and receiving help can make a difference to treatment outcome because (a) everyone is different, (b) there are effective treatment techniques and strategies that work, and (c) there is nothing to be lost by exploring what help might be right for you.

What sort of professional help is the most effective?

There are many forms of 'talking therapies' and you should ask your therapist or counsellor to describe and explain the type of therapy he or she offers, what it involves, how long it will last, and what the research evidence is for the type of technique or therapy he or she uses. Many types of therapy can be helpful, and talking to a therapist can be very helpful.

There is considerably less orthodoxy in the fields of counselling, psychotherapy, psychology, and psychiatry than in general medicine, where, for example, there is generally an agreement on the methods of treatment of many medical conditions, with minor differences in the application of treatment and management of the condition. However, when it comes to mental health, there is a greater variability on therapeutic methods and who offers which therapy. Counsellors, psychotherapists, psychologists, and psychiatrists are all involved in offering help, but each profession has its own language and way of thinking, and it can therefore be confusing. As a consequence, psychological/psychotherapeutic interventions can and do vary considerably, often depending on the type of approach the counsellor or therapist uses.

This then begs the question of which psychotherapeutic option is likely to be the most effective for PTSD. Whilst the contribution of psychoanalytic thinking to our understanding of the development PTSD should be acknowledged, there are no outcome studies to indicate the effectiveness of psychoanalytic or psychodynamic therapy for PTSD. In addition, despite the rapid growth in the number of counsellors, especially within primary care, there is little evidence that generic counselling, provided by itself, is particularly effective in the treatment of PTSD.

Often when someone is suffering from PTSD, and the situation is beginning to affect the individual's social and occupational functioning, more active, practical forms of intervention are helpful. Research suggests that a type of psychological therapy, known as CBT can be very effective. It is especially effective for the treatment of psychological trauma and for those individuals suffering from PTSD; this will be described in more detail later in the chapter.

Current treatment recommendations

The National Institute for Clinical Excellence in Health (NICE) in the UK is an independent organization responsible for providing national guidance and promoting good health and the treatment of specific clinical conditions. In addition, it produces clinical practice guidelines, derived from the best available research evidence, using predetermined and systematic methods to identify and evaluate all the evidence in relation to the specific condition in question. Where it is considered that this evidence is lacking, the guidelines aim to incorporate statements and recommendations based upon the consensus statements developed by the guidelines' group. The NICE guidelines, Post-traumatic Stress Disorder (PTSD): The Management of PTSD in Adults and Children in Primary and Secondary Care, were published in 2005 and were developed to advise on the treatment and management of PTSD. Guideline recommendations were developed by a multidisciplinary team of healthcare professionals, guideline methodologists, and PTSD sufferers, after consideration of the best available evidence. The intention is that these NICE guidelines (along with others) would be useful to clinicians and service commissioners in providing a high quality of care to PTSD sufferers, including emphasis on the importance of the experience of carers. The NICE guidelines are regularly updated, and the most recent update was in 2015.

The NICE guidelines for PTSD provide a comprehensive review on the current best practice in the assessment and management of PTSD in primary and secondary care. The intention is that once the national guidelines have been published and disseminated, local healthcare providers will be expected to produce plans and identify resources with its implementation along with appropriate timetables. The intention is that multidisciplinary health groups, involving commissioners, specialist mental health professionals, patients, and carers would undertake the translation of the implementation to local protocols. Ultimately, the nature and time frame of any local plans reflect upon local needs and the nature of existing provisions.

Trauma-focused psychological therapy

The NICE guidelines recommend that PTSD sufferers should be offered a course of trauma-focused psychological therapy; typically, this would mean trauma-focused CBT, which may often include EMDR (described below) and other techniques. CBT is conducted over a relatively short space of time, usually 8–12 individual treatment sessions, over a period of months. It is an active and directive form of therapy, aimed at teaching individuals how to confront and eventually overcome their fears, avoidances, and anxious thoughts. All cognitive behavioural methods are:

◆ Structured and directive in nature.

◆ Problem and technique orientated.

◆ Directed towards helping individuals achieve their goals.

◆ Collaborative.

◆ Focused on the 'here and now'.

◆ Based upon use of explicit, agreed treatment strategies.

Techniques also include helping the sufferer challenge and change problematic thoughts and meanings about the trauma, which may include feelings of guilt or loss of trust in others. CBT also includes exposure therapy. Exposure therapy helps the individual confront feared reminders and memories of the trauma in a graded way (i.e. taking a step at a time). Like any form of therapy, it can be challenging because the individual will have to confront situations they have been avoiding, often for a considerable time. It is a very human response to want to avoid pain at any cost, whether physical or emotional. Exposure to reminders and memories can be painful, but with help, encouragement, and support, many PTSD sufferers can come to terms with traumatic experiences.

Pierre Janet's (1909) therapeutic approach to traumatized patients was the first attempt to create a systematic, phase-orientated treatment of post-traumatic stress. Janet viewed the trauma response as a disorder of memory that interfered with effective action. He also believed, and taught, that effective treatment consisted of the importance of forming a stable therapeutic relationship, which would facilitate the retrieving and transforming of traumatic memories into meaningful experiences and taking effective action to overcome learned helplessness. Janet's belief that a good, safe therapeutic relationship—what he described as a 'rapport' between patient and therapist—was indispensable for resolution of the trauma. Whilst not everyone may achieve resolution of all their difficulties, his thinking about therapeutic relationships remains relevant today.

CBT

Exposure to reminders and memories of the trauma remain common to most approaches, but in CBT, exposure is conducted in a systematic way, based upon research that these approaches can be effective. Different aspects of CBT approaches to trauma are described next.

Assessment

Assessment is an extremely important process before therapy begins, and some of the areas that are addressed in assessment are covered in Chapter 3. However, in addition to the assessment interview, patients are also asked to fill in self-report questionnaires, which also provide very helpful information and are used to form a baseline and monitor progress, either session by session or at the end of therapy and at follow-up. These are relatively straightforward to fill out, and if there is any difficulty, ask a relative, friend, or the therapist to help. They provide a snapshot of specific aspects of the individual's traumatic experience, such as avoidance, mood, sleep, concentration, and the frequency of intrusive thoughts. The most common are described below, but there are others that may be used by the therapist to highlight or focus on areas they feel may be of benefit in therapy; one such example is the Psychological Well-being Post-Trauma Changes Questionnaire (PWB-PTCQ), which we have developed to assess changes in self-acceptance, autonomy, mastery, purpose in life, relationships, and personal growth (see Box 10.1). This is a short, easy-to-use tool that therapists may find useful alongside the more traditional measures of post-traumatic stress, to which we will now turn.

Interviews

The clinician-administered PTSD scale DSM IV

The clinician-administered PTSD scale (CAPS) for DSM IV is a well-validated instrument that is seen as a 'gold standard' diagnostic tool. It was developed to measure cardinal and hypothesized signs and symptoms of PTSD (Blake et al. 1995). It is not a self-report measure but is carried out as an interview by the therapist with the patient. The interview can be a lengthy process, taking over an hour to complete. It provides a method to evaluate the frequency and intensity of individual symptoms, as well as the impact of symptoms in social and occupational functioning, the overall intensity of the symptoms, and the validity of the ratings obtained. It also provides an opportunity for the clinician to rate the veracity and accuracy of symptom descriptions and their severity and intensity, thus allowing the overall validity of responses to be assessed. Factors considered are compliance with the interview, mental state (e.g. problems with concentration, comprehension of items, disassociation, and any evidence of efforts to exaggerate or minimize symptoms). Every symptom is rated for frequency (from 0 = never to 4 = daily or almost every day) and intensity (from 0 = none to 4 = extreme, incapacitating distress). Where a symptom is positively endorsed, the patient is asked to give a detailed description or example. The time frame used in the CAPS is a month period before the interview. The CAPS may often be used if individuals are attending for a medicolegal interview (i.e. they are being assessed for a litigation claim following a road-traffic collision or industrial injury). It is not used by all therapists but is often used in specialist treatment centres.

Self-report questionnaires

Some common self-report questionnaires are listed below. Unlike the CAPS, these questionnaires do not diagnose someone as having PTSD and they are not intended nor should they be used for this purpose. The list provided in the chapter is not meant as an exhaustive list, but merely as an indication of those in most frequent use.

Impact of event scale

The impact of event scale (IES) is widely used in research and clinical practice following exposure to traumatic events and is a measure of subjective distress in relation to the experience. It has 15 items and two subscales: intrusion/re-experiencing and avoidance. The usual 'cut-off' point is 35. This means that if a person scores 35 or more, they can be seen as having a significant reaction in the moderate-to-severe range (Horowitz et al. 1979).

For those that wish additionally to assess the hyper-arousal criteria of PTSD, there is also the revised impact of event scale (IES-R), which has 22 items that include feeling constantly on guard, irritability, and anger. Both versions of the IES are in common use (Horowitz et al. 1979).

The post-traumatic diagnostic scale

The post-traumatic diagnostic scale (PDS) enquires about PTSD symptoms and is designed to aid in diagnosis based on DSM-IV criteria. It gives a measure of PTSD symptom severity. The PDS offers respondents a checklist of 12 traumatic events. First, they have to endorse all those events that they have experienced and define which event has caused them the most distress. Second, respondents then rate each of 17 items corresponding to the 17 DSM-IV symptoms of PTSD. Each of the 17 items is rated on a four-point scale. Finally, respondents are asked questions regarding the duration of symptoms and inquiries regarding impairment in a variety of areas. Like other questionnaires, it is intended to be used in conjunction with a clinical interview and thorough assessment (Foa 1996).

Posttraumatic Avoidance Scale

Avoidance is a key factor. The Posttraumatic Avoidance Scale is a 20-item self-report measure of avoidance that has two ten-item subscales: (1) controlled avoidance (the degree to which people engage in efforts themselves to avoid reminders; e.g. Do you deliberately do things to stop yourself thinking about the event?), and (2) automatic avoidance (the degree to which people are avoidant involuntarily, such as emotional numbing; e.g. When you go over the event, does it feel like your emotions have been switched off?). The advantage of this measure is that it allows researchers and clinicians to explore these two different forms of avoidance. Each item is rated on a five-point scale, from never = 0 to always = 4 (Andrews et al. 2012).

Post-Traumatic Cognitions Inventory

The Post-Traumatic Cognitions Inventory questionnaire attempts to assess particular themes related to the individual's negative beliefs about the self, the world and self-blame. In the clinical setting, an individual's thoughts and beliefs can be focused on in treatment, and progress and outcome can be tracked over time (Foa et al.1999).

Psychological Well-Being—Post-Traumatic Changes Questionnaire

The Psychological Well-Being—Post-Traumatic Changes Questionnaire (PWB-PTCQ) is designed to assess people's views of themselves and how they have changed for the better or for the worse in relation to their psychological well-being in the aftermath of adversity. It is an 18-item (e.g. 'I have a sense of purpose in life.') self-report questionnaire that is designed to assess change on six domains: self-acceptance, autonomy, purpose in life, relationships, sense of mastery, and personal growth. Respondents are asked to rate how much they feel they have changed since the trauma. Each item is rated on a five-point scale, from 1 = 'much less so now' to 5 = 'much more so now' (Joseph et al. 2012).

Beck Depression Inventory

The Beck Depression Inventory is a well-known and well-validated clinical and research tool. It is a 21-item, self-rating questionnaire, allowing for rapid assessment of depressive symptoms. Sometimes it is administered on a weekly basis (Beck et al. 1988).

General Health Questionnaire-28

The General Health Questionnaire-28 (GHQ-28) is a self-rating screening tool for psychiatric problems in the general population. The threshold/cut-off point for identifying 'psychiatric caseness' (i.e. the likelihood that the individual could be classified as having minor mental health problems) is 5; however, if used with someone who has had a physical injury or has problems that are more complex, it would be more appropriate to raise the threshold/cut-off point to 13 or above (Goldberg 1981).

Posttraumatic Growth Inventory

Posttraumatic Growth Inventory (PTGI) is a 21-item (e.g. 'I have a greater appreciation for the value of my own life.') self-report questionnaire that is designed to assess perceptions of change on five subscales: new possibilities, personal strength, spiritual change, appreciation of life, and relating to others. Respondents are asked to rate their responses on a six-point Likert scale, and scores range from 0 = 'I did not change as a result of the event I described' to 5 = 'I changed to a very great degree as a result of the event I described.' We will return to the topic of post-traumatic growth in Chapter 10 (Tedeschi and Calhoun 1996).

Cognitive therapy

Cognitive therapy operates on a multilayered understanding of the relationships among cognitions (thoughts), behaviours, emotions, and how these are affected and influenced by an individual's experience; hence, it is described as a form of CBT, as thoughts, attitudes, and beliefs (i.e. attitudinal change) can only be brought about through behavioural experience. The model is problem-orientated, and it focusses on the 'here and now', is active, directive, and, most importantly, collaborative. The emphasis here is on the identification of the shattered beliefs and assumptions, and the rebuilding of these through what is described as 'cognitive restructuring'; in other words, trying to help individuals think differently about the experience and develop new meanings. Trauma-focused cognitive therapy attempts to change problematic meanings of the traumatic experience, such as 'What happened shows that I am bad/inferior/ useless person' and 'I cannot trust anyone anymore', and changing problematic coping responses, such as thought suppression, ruminating on negative outcomes, or selectively attending to threat.

Graded Exposure

Graded Exposure, also known as exposure *in vivo* (or real life), involves exposure in real life to feared/avoided situations, either directly related to the traumatic event or that resemble it in some way. This could be either graded or prolonged, and either therapist-aided or unaccompanied. Partners or significant-other family members are often encouraged to act as a co-therapist, if possible. Patients are given specific instructions and guidelines for exposure therapy, emphasis being placed on consistency within the treatment programme. A rationale for exposure is often given as follows:

Usually, some anxiety occurs when you start this type of programme. This is actually an important part of treatment, because often people think that the anxiety will continue and become intolerable. One of the valuable things you learn through treatment is that the anxiety does not increase to intolerable levels and it often subsides more rapidly than you might expect. Sometimes, anxiety starts to reduce within 20 minutes; more usually, half an hour to an hour. Another important thing that you will notice is that, after you have done exposure two or three times, the amount of discomfort you get at first becomes less and less. This is the best indication of how the treatment is working; as time goes on, you will find you will be able to do the exposure in this way and get no discomfort at all.

One way of describing the way exposure works, is to consider it a form of 'emotional physiotherapy'. For example, if a person has an accident and injures or breaks a limb, they are often prescribed a course of physiotherapy, which they have to attend regularly, and it is often painful, sometimes causing some discomfort for some hours afterwards, perhaps even a few days. When done in frequent, regular, and repeated sessions, there is a cumulative effect, and the distress and discomfort gradually decrease in time. In addition, exercises are also recommended and suggested. In this way, individuals gradually learn to use their limbs again. Experience of a case on the burns unit is a good illustration of this idea of emotional physiotherapy.

Another exposure-based therapy, which has been developed for use in different cultural contexts, is Narrative Exposure Therapy. It has been developed for use in a wide range of settings (e.g. refugee camps), and there is a strong evidence base to say that it is not only an effective approach to trauma treatment but also useful to great effect by lay therapists such as teachers and social workers (see Chapter 7, on Cultural Responses).

⑤ Chen's story

Chen was a man of Chinese origin, who was receiving treatment on the burns unit after being badly injured in an explosion in a holiday apartment. He spoke almost no English, but communicated through his wife, who spoke limited English, and his son, who was born in the UK. After leaving, he was attended for physiotherapy and occupational therapy (OT) regularly for his injuries. He was attending the OT department because his hands were badly injured. One day he attended the department as usual but found that the doors were being repaired and he would have to enter via the OT kitchen. This caused him to become extremely agitated and distressed, and, on discussions with his son, it transpired that he was extremely avoidant of the kitchen at home. The family ran a small takeaway restaurant, and Chen had often been responsible for most of the cooking before his accident.

The family reported that he was avoiding the kitchen in the family home because of all the traumatic reminders and triggers present (e.g. the cooker and sockets). In view of this, it was decided to try to attempt a Graded Exposure programme with him, starting in the OT kitchen and then at home. However, a meeting (including his wife and son) with his occupational therapist, physiotherapist, keyworker, and CBT therapist to explain and give a rationale of why this would help soon ran into problems as it became very difficult to explain the principles of the technique to Chen. After much discussion and several failed attempts to explain this, the CBT therapist decided to use the similarities between Graded Exposure and his regular physiotherapy. His son explained this to Chen and his wife, and after some animated discussion between them, they both began smiling and nodding. When asked by the team what had happened, his son said that Chen's wife had told him this was to be 'physiotherapy for his heart', a concept he clearly understood and identified with—hence, the term *emotional physiotherapy*!

Exposure may involve revisiting the site or scene of the traumatic event. This can be extremely important, if it is possible and safe to do so. This allows the person to discriminate 'then' versus 'now' and to develop new meanings about the experience. This should only be attempted at a safe point in therapy and should be therapist-aided, as new meanings may emerge that will need to be addressed in treatment.

To emphasize the importance and value of real-life exposure, we need to revisit Jill's experience after surviving a rail disaster (in Chapter 3). Whilst she found the early counselling helpful, she found it did not address the significant issues of avoidance, which were seriously affecting her ability to work, as well as affecting her social and family life. Her experience of exposure also helped her overcome her many anxieties following her involvement in a rail disaster.

📖 Jill's story (continued)

Later, I changed to a different therapist to focus on rolling back my avoidance behaviours. Initially, I had two sessions of EMDR, which made a difference to anxiety when anticipating rail travel, but I also found the CBT and exposure therapy very beneficial. Under guidance from my therapist, I drew up, and followed diligently, a timetable for gradual exposure. It began with building up resilience to driving, through more consistent exposure (which I was also avoiding), then sitting on train platforms, watching trains, building up to repeated train journeys on slow then high-speed trains, over a 6-month period.

I also developed mantras/prayers and creative thought patterns to help me cope with my wider range of anxieties. Eighteen months (and about ten sessions) after beginning the therapy, I feel I am about 75% back to normal with regard to travelling by train and have strategies to help me cope when feeing vulnerable. I am now far more reflective about the train crash and think of it as being more in the past than in the present. I have even recently travelled by air, something I had been dreading!

Exposure in imagination

This involves the patients being asked to relive their traumatic memories, in the first person and present tense, and giving as much detail as possible about the traumatic event and their thoughts, emotions, and responses; attention would be paid to specific aspects (e.g. smell and sounds). Often it is possible to construct a hierarchy, using material that is less distressing first. At the top of the hierarchy are those aspects of the traumatic event that are most upsetting, and at the bottom, the least-upsetting aspects. Imaginal exposure involves persons working their way up the hierarchy in their imagination, beginning with the least-upsetting aspects. Persons engage in imagination with their experience until it no longer upsets them. They then move on to the next upsetting aspects and repeat the exercise. At specific points a rewind and hold technique is used, whereby they are asked to concentrate on the worst aspect of the traumatic event, to freeze and hold the image, whilst repeatedly describing in detail all they can remember about this element of the trauma. This is repeated until habituation occurs. The session is audiotaped, and they are asked to practise this between sessions, until habituation occurs; a 50%–70% reduction in anxiety is desirable for effective reduction in symptoms. As with any exposure therapy, consistency and regular practice is essential. However, the last decade has seen a number of developments in our thinking about the nature of traumatic memories, and, subsequently, approaches that are more sophisticated and based on similar ideas have been developed, such as 'imagery rescripting'. EMDR has tended to become the 'technique of choice' over the past 2 decades, and many therapists may favour this approach over imaginal-exposure techniques.

Imagery rescripting is primarily an experiential technique where the patients are encouraged to think of their problematic and intrusive memories as 'ghosts from the past'. Interestingly, Pierre Janet described examples of 'imagery substitution' in 1889 in his book *L'Automatisme Psychologique*, which mirror the techniques discussed here. The treatment may be roughly explained as follows:

Traumatic events may leave us with distressing images and memories that haunt us and colour our experience of the present. Sometimes these disturbing and upsetting memories are stored with the meanings they had at the time of the event and we think they say a lot about the kind of person we are. Some of these beliefs may be unhelpful, distorted, out of proportion, and no longer valid or true. These memories need to be updated so that they take their proper place in amongst your other memories. The most effective way of doing this is to get at the memories by re-experiencing them in your imagination. We can then try to transform the memories by reflecting on their meanings and using imagery that is more creative, so they become less distressing.

Common questions during this process may be as follows:

- Is the image you experience based on an actual event?

- What would happen if you allowed the image to continue?

- Can you visualize yourself today, having survived the event, entering the scene?

- Where are you, and what do you see?

- What would the scene look like projected onto a cinema screen or seen from a moving train?

◆ Imagine watching the image on TV and then switching it off, making it smaller, further away, dimmer ... freeze the image, make it black and white.

Length of such sessions should be 60–90 minutes, and it is important not rush imagery work; several sessions may be needed to deal with one specific memory. There are, therefore, occasions where sessions of CBT may exceed the 8–12 sessions, especially in more complex presentations, as in the following case example using EMDR.

EMDR

The EMDR technique is often included as part of CBT. EMDR can be effective in dealing with many trauma symptoms. This is not a 'stand-alone' technique, and it should be used as part of the course of CBT. EMDR is a relatively new and effective treatment for PTSD, as well as other clinical conditions.

EMDR literally owes its beginnings to a walk in the park. The founder of EMDR, Francine Shapiro, wrote that EMDR was based on a serendipitous discovery made in May 1987. She described that whilst walking through a park, she noticed that she was troubled by some disturbing thoughts, which 'suddenly disappeared'. She also noted that when she tried to recall these thoughts, they were not as disturbing or as valid as they had been previously. She postulated that upsetting thoughts in general had a repetitive quality to them, which only change if the individual does something to stop or change them. However, Shapiro noted that the disturbing thoughts were changing without conscious effort. After paying close attention to this phenomenon, she noticed that during her walk, her eyes had moved from side to side and she speculated that this might have been a key factor in her ability to process the disturbing memories. After experimentation with over 70 subjects, she published the first paper on EMDR in 1989.

In essence, EMDR involves pairing memories/disturbing thoughts and the resultant emotions with repeated saccadic (rapid and rhythmic) eye movements, resulting in the desensitization, or reduction in distress caused by the memories. In patients unable to use eye movements, other bi-lateral stimuli, such as hand taps, are used. Hand taps are also used when applying the technique with children, especially younger children, where language may be a problem. A similar pairing of memory and chosen positive cognitions or rational self-statements, with further eye movements (or chosen stimuli), constitutes the reprocessing component (Shapiro and Forrest, 1997). The therapist will ask about changes during the process of EMDR and some of these may be as follows:

◆ Have you noticed the image change at all?

◆ Has it become blurred, sharper, and more vivid?

- Has it moved farther away?
- Has it changed colour?
- What appears different, if anything?
- What bodily changes do you notice, compared with when we started?
- Has your anxiety reduced, remained the same, or gotten worse?

It is often seen as being most useful with what is described as single-episode trauma (e.g. the road-traffic collision or an assault) but has often been used successfully with longer term accumulative trauma, such as sexual abuse, as illustrated by Sam's story.

📄 Sam's story

Sam is 32 years old. She has eight siblings in total: three male and five female. Six are stepsiblings by marriage. Both mother and father had previous marriages with the father having four previous children (two male and two female) and the mother two (female). The mother and father came together, producing three further children, with Sam being the second to the youngest. Sam's eldest sibling is her 45-year-old stepsister.

Sam's father was a paedophile and he abused, both physically and sexually, all nine children in varying degrees. Sam's first memory of being abused by her father was around the age of 3 years and the latest at 7 years. Her father also allowed other adult males to abuse Sam sexually. She had an awareness of the sexual abuse to some of her siblings.

Approximately 5 years ago, Sam experienced a crisis and suffered a severe bout of depression. She attended a sexual abuse support group for a year and received one-to-one counselling for a further 6 months. Sam was referred for CBT. She received over 20 sessions of CBT, including EMDR. After the EMDR sessions and when evaluating her therapeutic experience, she reported:

All I can say is that I have reached a place within myself that I have never been able to before this. I was sceptical and not sure whether it was just the right time, the therapy or a combination of both, but EMDR seems to have 'shifted' something. I think its strength of belief. It's as though the pain and shit beliefs I've carried all my life about myself have been put down, as though I've finally been able to separate, accept, let go and even, who knows, forgive? Suppose it's just a process really. I've finally been able to make the steps to move on and can't wait to grab the life I now feel is ahead of me.

EMDR was a controversial technique amongst the psychology and psycho-therapy community when first used, but it is now well established and used by many therapists working with trauma survivors. The precise mechanism for clinically reported change remains unclear, but it has been and continues to be the subject of considerable ongoing research. While there is a growing body of scientific literature on the technique, and a number of studies confirm the effectiveness of EMDR in the treatment of PTSD, this does not prove Shapiro's idea that it is because of eye movements. Critics have suggested that EMDR works, not because of anything to do with eye movements but because it involves exposure. However, even if the technique does not work with every-one, it is effective with many trauma survivors. EMDR also needs to be used with careful assessment, and attention needs to be paid to the meaning of the traumatic experience as the specifics of the traumatic event itself. EMDR is often used as part of the CBT repertoire by many therapists, whilst some per-ceive it to be a therapy in its own right. There is no 'right' or 'wrong' way, but as with any psychological technique, there needs to be a judicious, considered use of the technique rather than a mechanistic and simplistic application of the process.

Medication and drug treatments

Out of the mental health professions, it is only psychiatrists who are permit-ted to prescribe medication. Some nurses (nurse prescribers) can prescribe medication, but this is rarer in mental health. The NICE guidelines do not recommend medication as a first-line treatment for PTSD. Pharmacological treatments in PTSD sufferers is often considered a critical component of treatment, but it should proceed with a careful and well-thought-out plan, which should be monitored by the therapist, GP, and any other mental health professional involved. The most common medications used for PTSD, as an adjunct to psychological therapy, are the selective serotonin reuptake inhibi-tors. These are usually anti-depressants, some of which are commonly used for PTSD sufferers.

Common concerns of PTSD sufferers about taking medication, such as fears of addiction or of taking medication will be seen as a weakness, should be addressed in early discussions about prescribing options. All patients who are prescribed anti-depressants should be informed, at the time that treatment is started, of potential side effects and the risk of sudden discon-tinuation/withdrawal. The onset of discontinuation/withdrawal symptoms is usually within 5 days of stopping the drug. Generally, anti-depressant drugs recommended for use in PTSD should be discontinued over at least a 4-week period, although some people will require longer periods. Written information should be made available, if possible. The most com-mon side effects are nausea, diarrhoea, abdominal discomfort, and sexual dysfunction.

Other therapies

Other therapies are designed to help people make sense of their experiences, to confront the existential issues, and to make new meanings. Existential and humanistic therapists can offer people valuable help in working through trauma and what it means to them and in rebuilding their lives. Like CBT, these are also talking therapies, with the difference being that the therapist will be less concerned with assessment, diagnosis, and offering a treatment. Rather, the therapist is concerned to understand how you, the client, see things. The therapist wants to understand how it is for you, and to help you make sense of things in your own time and in your own way. The therapist also wants to understand the meaning of the experience for the individual and help them make sense of it. It is up to the individuals to decide what is right for them at the point in their lives; they decide to seek help and determine what their priorities and goals are at that time. Existential and humanistic therapists will emphasize the choices people have and their own responsibility to shape their own lives (Joseph, 2004).

Most therapists will offer a tailored approach to therapy, which will help to address the client's unique situation. For example, therapists may encourage people to become more mindful, which may help them deal with stress, or become compassionate towards themselves if they are overly self-critical.

These therapies can be extremely valuable at the right time in a person's life. But as we have seen, avoidance is a big problem with people following trauma; hence, it may be hard for people to engage with existential and humanistic therapies until they are willing to confront their experiences. Some of the treatments for PTSD can therefore be useful to pave the way for these other therapies, which help some people to want to explore deeper meanings of their experiences. For many, trauma-focused CBT will be effective not only in dealing with PTSD symptoms, but also with issues of guilt and shame. As we will see in Chapter 10, trauma can often be a turning point in people's lives, and, as such, good therapists will help individuals to find meaning and renegotiate their priorities in light of their traumatic experience, whatever therapy they practise.

The impact of litigation on the course of treatment and recovery

One issue that often affects trauma survivors is litigation, especially following road-traffic collisions and industrial injury. There have also been many high-profile compensation cases concerning veterans and individuals who have developed a medical condition or suffered an injury or loss as a result of medical negligence. While it is appropriate in many cases for people to seek compensation for psychological suffering, this can be problematic in its own right. It is often the case that medicolegal processes, which can be protracted and complicated, serve to prolong people's distress. It is the exception rather than the rule that individuals 'invent' their symptoms and are driven by the anticipated financial rewards.

Most medicolegal cases seen by the vast majority of psychologists, psychotherapists, psychiatrists, and other mental health professionals, are genuine. If, for example, anyone is involved in a road-traffic collision or industrial accident that was caused by someone else and liability is admitted, then the individual is legitimately entitled to compensation through the other party's insurance. This can be for either physical or psychiatric injury. The amount of compensation is calculated by reference to a variety of factors (e.g. loss of earnings, the nature of damage or injury, the impact on social and occupational functioning, and costs of treatments for physical or psychological care). Claimants are advised as to the amount they may be entitled to by their legal representatives; they do not—contrary to popular belief—decide upon the amount themselves. There is also little or no evidence for what is known as 'compensation neuroses'. This is when persons are seen to be exaggerating or prolonging their symptoms and the impact this has on their lives in order to gain a greater financial settlement. Previous studies of victims of road-traffic collisions or accidental injury have shown that symptoms do not disappear or improve when the legal process has ended. Of course, there are always individual examples that could be cited to the contrary, but these would be the exception rather than the rule.

There are concerns over compensation issues and subsequently the legitimacy, and possible overuse, of the PTSD diagnosis. However, we must be careful not to misrepresent the plight of those who have suffered a traumatic experience through the fault or negligence of others. The medicolegal process can be a difficult and unpleasant experience that many individuals persevere with, not because they want financial rewards, but because they wish justice to be done. Before embarking on a course of action for medicolegal compensation, it is worth considering the following:

◆ The solicitor for the claimant usually obtains a medical report in the first instance, before the issue of any court proceedings, after agreeing the identity of the expert to be instructed with the other party's insurers or solicitor. However, if after considering the report the other party is unhappy with the findings in the report, then they may seek to obtain their own expert's report. For instance, the other party may seek to argue that pre-existing vulnerabilities are the prime cause of distress, rather than any psychiatric or psychological injury resulting from the accident. This can make Claimants feel that their honesty is being questioned in some way.

◆ Claimants often have to attend many appointments with what are known as 'expert witnesses'. These are professional experts in their field in either physical medicine or mental health (e.g. orthopaedics, psychiatry, psychology, or other specialty).

- These appointments invariably involve travel, sometimes over long distances if the expert is not local. This in itself can be stressful, because it may involve the claimant (or their partner or relative) having time off from work, and it in itself may be financially costly.

- The assessments often, if not always, involve repeated telling of the story, sometimes in great detail.

- Under the court rules, the solicitors for each party can agree to appoint what is known as a joint expert, which means that both parties agree to be bound by the single expert's opinion however favourable or unfavourable that may be. This has the benefit of removing the need for a person to see more than one expert in each speciality but it is not always appropriate in all cases.

- Under the law the burden is on the injured party to prove fault, rather than the other party proving he or she is not at fault, which some people feel is unfair. This can enhance the sense of injustice they already feel.

- In cases where the other party denies any liability for the claimant's claim, court proceedings often have to be issued in order to progress matters, and ultimately the claimant may have to appear in court to give evidence in person. This is often a source of serious concern to an individual, which can compound his or her other problems. However, the majority of claims are settled out of court.

- Reports often take time to produce, and sometimes many weeks may elapse before the report is produced. However, it is the ethical responsibility of the expert to produce the report as soon as possible in order not to delay the process. This inevitably involves more delays as legal teams then have to consider what action needs to be taken in their client's best interest and the financial implications. Medicolegal reports should ideally be produced as soon as possible after the assessment, but a reasonable time frame should be within 2 to 3 weeks of the assessment date.

- If recommendations for treatment are made, then applications for funding have to be made in order to facilitate that, as most of these treatments, whilst available under the NHS, may involve long waiting lists, and, therefore, private treatment is often sought.

- The majority of compensation payments are not large. Sums of six or seven figures are rare but are more likely to be in the tens of thousands. Large compensation payments are usually made when there is a loss of life, limb, or the person needs long-term treatment or care (e.g. following a head or spinal injury).

- Compensation for criminal injuries are most often made through the Criminal Injuries Compensation Authority, and, again, these sums are not vast and are awarded on a tariff system for injuries, which many victims see as unfair. However, there is an appeals process in place for those who contest their awards.

♦ Any payments made before a final settlement, known as 'interim payments' (e.g. for the cost of travel, subsistence, any preliminary treatments, investigations, and assessments) are deducted from the final settlement to avoid 'double recovery' under the law, something many are not aware of, as it is often not made explicit. Therefore, these issues should be discussed with the legal representative.

It must be noted that the laws surrounding compensation for psychiatric injury will differ between countries, and there are differences in the UK between Scottish and English law. This will also differ in other countries.

Conclusion

Therapeutic approaches, such as CBT, including techniques like EMDR, have been demonstrated to be effective with PTSD sufferers: these approaches work by facilitating a constructive engagement with their fears, avoidances, and shattered assumptions about themselves, others, and the world, enabling survivors to develop new meanings and make sense of their experience. Other therapies, such as existential and humanistic therapies, can also be helpful in providing an opportunity for people to confront any existential issues they may be struggling with. These forms of therapy are less directive in nature. They may often be helpful to those people who want to explore issues and experiences that they feel have been brought to the fore as a direct or indirect result of the traumatic event. It must be emphasized that different therapies will suit different people and at different times in their lives. The individual needs to decide what is best suited to their circumstances, needs, and goals at the time they seek help.

References

Andrews, L., Joseph, S., Troop, N., Rooyen, T. V., Dunn, B. D, and Dalgleish, T. (2012). The structure of avoidance following trauma: development and validation of the Posttraumatic Avoidance Scale (PAS). *Traumatology* 19, 126–135.

Beck, A., Steer, R., and Garbin, M. (1988). Psychometric properties of the Beck Depression Inventory: twenty-five years of evaluation. *Journal of Clinical Psychology Review* 8, 77–100.

Blake, D. D., Weathers, F. W., Nagy, L. M., Kaloupek, D. G., Gusman, F. D., Charney, D. S., and Keane, T. M. (1995). The development of a clinician-administered PTSD scale. *Journal of Traumatic Stress* 8, 75–90.

Brewin, C., Scragg, P., Robertson, M., et al. (2008). Promoting mental health following the London bombings: a screen and treat approach. *Journal of Traumatic Stress* 21(1) 3–8.

Foa, E. B. (1996). *Posttraumatic stress diagnostic scale (PDS)*. Minneapolis: National Computer Systems.

Foa, E. B., Ehlers, A., Clark, D. M., Tolin, D. F., and Orsillo, S. M. (1999). The Posttraumatic Cognitions Inventory (PTCI): development and validation. *Psychological Assessment* 11(3), 303–314.

Goldberg, D. (1981). *General health questionnaire.* Berkshire: NFER-NELSON.

Horowitz, M., Wilner, N., and Alvarez, W. (1979). Impact of event scale: a measure of subjective stress. *Psychosomatic Medicine 41*(3), 209–218.

Janet, P. (1909). *Les névroses.* Paris: Flammarion.

Joseph, S., Maltby, J., Wood, A. M., Stockton, H., Hunt, N., and Regel, S. (2012). The psychological well-being – post –traumatic changes questionnaire (PWB_PTCQ): reliability, validity, and psychological trauma. *Theory, Research, Practice and Policy 4*, 420–428.

Joseph, S. (2004). Client–centred therapy, post–traumatic stress disorder and post-traumatic growth: Theoretical perspectives and practical implications. *Psychology and Psychotherapy: Theory, Research and Practice 77*(1), 101–119.

National Institute for Clinical Excellence (NICE). (2005). *Post-traumatic stress disorder (PTSD): the management of PTSD in adults and children in primary and secondary care.* London: Gaskell. (www.nice.org.uk).

Shapiro, F. (1989). Efficacy of the eye movement desensitization procedure in the treatment of traumatic memories. *Journal of Traumatic Stress 2*, 199–233.

Shapiro, F., and Forrest, M. S. (1997). EMDR: *the breakthrough therapy for overcoming anxiety, stress and trauma.* New York: Basic Books.

Tedeschi, R. G., and Calhoun, L. G. (1996). The posttraumatic growth inventory: measuring the positive legacy of trauma. *Journal of Traumatic Stress 9*, 455–471.

10

Post-traumatic growth

> ## ➔ Key Points
>
> ◆ People often report perceiving benefits following trauma, a phenomena referred to as post-traumatic growth.
>
> ◆ Frequently, people mention improved relationships, changes in life philosophy, and shifts in how they think about themselves.
>
> ◆ Post-traumatic growth arises from the struggle to make sense of what has happened.
>
> ◆ Post-traumatic growth can help people cope.
>
> ◆ Therapists can help people to explore post-traumatic growth.
>
> ◆ Post-traumatic growth may lead to reductions in post-traumatic stress.

Introduction

Throughout human history, literature, religions, and philosophies have conveyed the idea that there are benefits to be found following exposure to adversity, extreme stress, and trauma. Post-traumatic growth (PTG) is the term coined by Richard Tedeschi and Lawrence Calhoun in the mid 1990s to describe the benefits that are often reported by survivors of trauma (Tedeschi and Calhoun 1996). Initially there was some debate and controversy over the idea of PTG. But there is now convincing research evidence that people often experience PTG leading to new developments in clinical practice and self-help strategies for survivors.

PTG refers, not just to recovery following stressful and traumatic events, but how events can sometimes serve as the springboard to a higher level of psychological well-being. Like trees caught in a wind, which immediately spring back to their original shape when the wind dies down, some people quickly recover from trauma. That is what we mean by recovery. The idea of PTG is different to the idea of recovery.

In contrast, in a massive wind, the branches of trees will break, and their limbs will be twisted out of shape. Those trees don't bounce back to their original shape. That is more like what happens following trauma. People are so overwhelmed by what happens to them that they are permanently changed. As we have seen in the previous chapters, trauma can be deeply distressing, but PTG research has also shown that sometimes the ways that people are affected can be life changing in positive ways that lead to enhanced psychological well-being.

Three broad but related dimensions of benefit finding have been described. First, relationships are enhanced in some way; for example, that people now value their friends and family more and feel an increased compassion and kindness towards others. Second, people change their views of themselves in some way; for example, that they have a greater sense of personal resiliency, wisdom, and strength, perhaps coupled with a greater acceptance of their vulnerabilities and limitations. Third, there are reports of changes in life philosophy; for example, finding a fresh appreciation for each new day and shifts in understanding of what really matters in life (Joseph 2013). For example, for Karen, a survivor of childhood abuse, it was the recognition that change is inevitable, being able to accept the past and live in the present: "I know though that life is change and one of the ways I have changed is a much greater sense of living in the present, being present now and accepting that everything changes ..." (quoted in Woodward and Joseph 2003, 279).

Living in the present was also mentioned by Isobella, who was bereaved of her husband. She described how she now views life as a positive learning process and is now more determined to be herself. However, she also adds that her biggest change is in her attitude to death: "I don't worry about silly things anymore, and if something is important to me I make an effort to do or say something about it. I speak my mind and have no regrets about anything ... The biggest thing I've gained from this is that I don't fear death ..." (quoted in Woodward and Joseph, 2003, 279).

Measuring positive change following trauma

Various psychological self-report tests have been developed to assess positive changes and personal growth following adversity. The most widely used measure is the Posttraumatic Growth Inventory (PTGI) mentioned previously in Chapter 9. Another is the more recently developed Psychological Well-Being—Post-Traumatic Changes Questionnaire (PWB-PTCQ; Joseph et al. 2012) (Box 10.1). The PWB-PTCQ is designed to assess people's views of themselves and how they have changed in the aftermath of adversity. It is an 18-item questionnaire that is designed to assess change on six domains: self-acceptance, autonomy, purpose in life, relationships, sense of mastery, and personal growth. The advantage of the PWB-PTCQ for therapists is that is provides clients with the opportunity to rate in what direction, either positive or negative, that their changes on each of these dimensions has been.

Box 10.1 Psychological Well-Being—Post-Traumatic Change Questionnaire (PWB-PTCQ)

Think about how you feel about yourself at the present time. Please read each of the following statements and rate how you have changed as a result of the trauma.

5 = Much more so now
4 = A bit more so now
3 = I feel the same about this as before
2 = A bit less so now
1 = Much less so now

_____ 1. I like myself.

_____ 2. I have confidence in my opinions.

_____ 3. I have a sense of purpose in life.

_____ 4. I have strong and close relationships in my life.

_____ 5. I feel I am in control of my life.

_____ 6. I am open to new experiences that challenge me.

_____ 7. I accept who I am, with both my strengths and limitations.

_____ 8. I don't worry what other people think of me.

_____ 9. My life has meaning.

_____ 10. I am a compassionate and giving person.

_____ 11. I handle my responsibilities in life well.

_____ 12. I am always seeking to learn about myself.

_____ 13. I respect myself.

_____ 14. I know what is important to me and will stand my ground, even if others disagree.

_____ 15. I feel that my life is worthwhile and that I play a valuable role in things.

_____ 16. I am grateful to have people in my life who care for me.

_____ 17. I am able to cope with what life throws at me.

_____ 18. I am hopeful about my future and look forward to new possibilities.

Add up your scores to all 18 statements. Scores over 54 indicate the presence of positive change. The maximum score is 90. The higher your score, the more positive change you have experienced.

You may have changed more on some areas than others. Self-acceptance (statements 1, 7, & 13), autonomy (statements 2, 8, & 14), purpose in life (statements 3, 9, & 15), relationships (statements 4, 10, & 16), sense of mastery (statements 5, 11, & 17), and personal growth (statements 6, 12, & 18).

Questionnaires like the PWB-PTCQ can be very useful to survivors of trauma in helping them to think about the ways in which their lives have changed. Therapists and clinicians may find it helpful to use the PWB-PTCQ alongside some of the other measures of post-traumatic stress that we mentioned in Chapter 9. Survivors who are deeply distressed may sometimes be surprised to discover the ways in which their lives have changed. This can fuel new strengths within them and ways of coping that help them deal with the challenges they are facing.

The amount of PTG that people experience varies between different research studies, depending on the types of groups studied, the context and experiences of those in the studies, and the type of research methods used. However, it would be expected that anywhere between 30% and 70% of people may typically experience some form of benefit following traumatic events. In one study, it was found that 58% of people in a national American survey reported benefits 2 months after the terrorist attacks in New York on 11 September 2001 (Poulin et al. 2009).

PTG does not mean that the person is no longer suffering from post-traumatic stress or the other problems they may be facing, but simply that trauma can have a wide range of effects. If we only focus on the negative consequences, we are missing out on the possibilities of positive change and their benefits for helping us cope.

As therapists ourselves, we are cautious about talking too much about PTG with our clients, certainly not in the early days following trauma. Positive changes are not usually reported in the very immediate aftermath but at some time later. In the immediate aftermath, people are confused and disorientated, and may be experiencing shock. In the subsequent weeks, they may be emotionally confused and experiencing post-traumatic stress. Until the person has reached a certain emotional equilibrium, it is likely to be too soon to think about PTG. For this reason, we would usually be careful about even introducing the topic of PTG to clients. What we find is that when the time is right for the person, they are likely to introduce the topic themselves, if we give them the space to do so.

As already mentioned, PTG is likely to be present alongside psychological distress. It is not that the experience of PTG is mutually exclusive to other more negative psychological consequences such as post-traumatic stress. In the early days, post-traumatic stress can be so overwhelming that people will be unlikely to experience PTG. But as time passes and the symptoms of post-traumatic stress abate to more tolerable levels, it seems that to some extent, it is the distress that helps to trigger the search for PTG. In fact, we have described how post-traumatic stress is the engine of PTG. And in turn, as people find PTG, this may help them to cope better with the distress.

📖 Anna's story

Anna is a 26-year-old woman who was the victim of a violent rape by four men, whilst on holiday on a Greek island. Stuart, her boyfriend, who was with her at the time, was also badly physically assaulted in the attack. The couple did report the assault, which was a high-profile case, making the national and international news. On return to the UK, Anna reported it to the British police and was subsequently seen by a forensic surgeon. She went through the normal process that many rape survivors have to undergo in the UK. She was persuaded to return to Greece to try to take the matter further, which she subsequently did but no one was arrested or charged with the assault. As can be expected, the return to the place of the assault was a significant retraumatizing factor for her.

In the months and years that followed, Anna developed significant symptoms of post-traumatic stress disorder and a prolonged period of depression. She had put on a significant amount of weight, increased her alcohol consumption, had given up her job, developed a range of avoidance behaviours, could not stay alone in the house, and had started sleeping with a carving knife under her pillow. By this time she had married Stuart, who had been supportive throughout. Their feelings for each other had not changed as a result of their experience: if anything, they had grown closer together. They eventually had a child and the subsequent birth of her daughter, Claire, prompted Anna to see her general practitioner, as she felt that she would not be able to look after her daughter, given the problems she was having, and this prompted her to seek treatment. A referral was subsequently made, and Anna received 14 sessions of trauma-focused cognitive behavioural therapy, which included eye movement desensitization and reprocessing (EMDR). She made significant progress and when seen at a 1-year follow-up appointment, she reported that she had made 90% improvement overall, was working, going out with friends on a regular basis, could stay alone at home when Stuart was working away, and had discontinued her antidepressants.

Whilst Anna's story is shocking and would affect anyone in similar circumstances, she worked hard to bring about change in her life, in order to improve the quality of her own life and that of her daughter and family. She realized she could not continue with her life the way she had been doing. There is, however, a further tragic postscript to her story, which could be seen as illustrative of PTG. Four years to the day following the assault, whilst on holiday with her family, Stuart literally dropped dead at the dining table at the holiday cottage on the second day of their holiday. Whilst Anna quite naturally experienced a traumatic bereavement, over the years, she has come through this, come to terms with Stuart's loss, and has remarried. Whilst this brief vignette does not do full justice to her story or her resourcefulness in the face of overwhelming adversity, the following quotes taken from an interview some years following Stuart's death are illuminating and could be seen as illustrative of PTG.

> ... what happened in Greece was such a huge trauma ... a huge thing—but I came through that and I thought after Greece I would never be able to live a normal life again ever. Then I was proved wrong because obviously with the stuff we did together I got my life back to normality and then, with Stuart dying, it gave me belief in myself that I could come through that, and it has also made me think that life's very short and we have got to make the most of what you've got....

> I think over the last year, obviously there have been changes and my whole outlook on life is different because I had always thought I would have a big family, and I know that has changed now, but I can accept that that is the way it is now. I think I don't look as far into the future now, I just take.... Not every day as it comes, but just take short periods of time to see what happens, rather than planning the future. I think that has changed me as a person.

> Sometimes I think—I really can't believe that I am in this point in my life, laughing and happy—and even when I got out of the car today and walked up to see you—it is a long way from the time when I first came to see you and can't believe I come on my own and I wondered myself how I cope. I came because I have to, because I feel I have no choice, because I have got Claire who has to be able to live her life happily, and I also feel now—and I didn't always feel like this—that life is for living and I have got no choice. I am here, so I can either enjoy it and get on with it or be miserable.

After Anna remarried, she had another child. She had a little boy, who, despite developing serious medical problems at birth, is now thriving.

Findings from the research on growth following adversity

Following the capsize of the Herald of Free Enterprise ferry in 1987, a survey of survivors asked them about the ways they had changed as a result of the accident (Joseph, Williams, and Yule 1993). Almost half of those surveyed reported positive changes in outlook, making statements such as:

- I don't take life for granted anymore.
- I value my relationships much more now.
- I'm a more understanding and tolerant person now.

Since this study, many others have reported PTG following a range of stressful and traumatic events, such as bereavement, accidents, disasters, chronic and life-threatening illness, abuse in childhood (sexual, physical, and emotional), sexual assault, and war and conflict.

Research has also begun to document why some people and not others are more likely to report PTG. Are some people more inclined to find benefits in their experience? The answer seems to be 'yes'. Studies of groups of people following adversity suggested that, while growth is not always reported by everyone, at least some people reported growth in all of the studies, suggesting that all life events have the potential to be triggers for positive change.

However, the main findings from research (see Helgeson, Reynolds, and Tomich 2006; Linley and Joseph 2004) are about what people bring to the situation themselves and what they do:

- Personality seems important. People who were more extraverted, open to experience, agreeable, conscientious, and emotionally stable, were more likely to report PTG.
- Optimistic people were more likely to report PTG.
- People who are more able to cope actively with problems in their life are more likely to experience PTG.
- People who were more able to deal with their emotions, such as by seeking out support from others, were more likely to report PTG.
- People who are able to use positive reinterpretation as a way of coping were more likely to report PTG.
- People who use more acceptance coping strategies were more likely to report PTG.
- People most likely to experience PTG have more nurturing, accepting, validating, and loving social relationships.

◆ But although some people seem to be more likely to find PTG than others, this does not mean that other people will not be able to. We can learn from those who do find benefits about what they do and use this knowledge to help others. People can be helped to develop their social support systems, cultivate new ways of coping, and become more optimistic in their outlook.

Considerations for therapy

Joseph, Murphy, and Regel (2012) use the psychosocial model described in Chapter 2 to describe points of clinical intervention to create and upwards and constructive positive cycle of change for clients.

Interventions may be directed at changing the social context, such as:

◆ Active, empathic listening

◆ Helping the client build social support in their lives

Provide opportunity for the client to confront their memories and reassess the meanings and significance of the event:

◆ Engage the client in exposure-related activities

◆ Promote reappraisal of the event, its meaning, and its significance in the client's life

◆ Help to normalize distressing emotional states

Help clients learn new coping skills and build positive emotions:

◆ Promote helpful coping strategies

◆ Promote positive emotional states

Therapists can provide such help, which can not only reduce the symptoms of post-traumatic stress but may also lead to the client developing an upwards and constructive cycle as new coping behaviours lead to more optimistic outlooks and positive psychological states, eventually resulting in deep-seated changes in personality that can be described as PTG.

In our own work, we have emphasized that growth following adversity is a normal and natural process, one that people are innately motivated towards. The task of the therapist is not to supply people with the answers to their questions and tell them what meaning to find in their experience. People will do this for themselves. The task is to provide the safe, supportive opportunity for this to take place.

Experimental studies to test whether the principles of growth might somehow be introduced as part of a clinical intervention are encouraging. For example, a study that randomly assigned breast cancer patients to one of two groups, either to write about the facts of the cancer experience or to write about their positive thoughts and feelings regarding the experience, found that those assigned to write about positive experiences had significantly fewer medical appointments for cancer-related problems 3months later (Stanton et al. 2002). Therapists should be aware of the potential for positive change in their clients following stress and trauma.

But it must also be recognized that adversity does not lead to positive change for everyone. Therefore, therapists need to be careful not to inadvertently imply that clients have in some way failed by not making more of their experience, or that there is anything inherently positive in their experience. PTG should be viewed as originating not from the event but from within the individuals themselves, through the process of their struggle with the event and its aftermath.

There is also much that people can do for themselves or a family member, as we will discuss in Chapter 11.

PTG seems to have implications for health and well-being. One important example is the groundbreaking work of Glenn Affleck and colleagues (1987), who found that perceived benefits at 7 weeks following a heart attack significantly predicted less chance of a heart attack recurrence and lower general health problems 8 years later, when patients were followed-up. Other studies since have also shown that those who experience PTG are less likely to have problems of depression, anxiety, and post-traumatic stress subsequently.

Turning to theory, Calhoun and Tedeschi (2012), the pioneers of this area of research, suggest that traumatic events serve as significant challenges by shattering prior goals and beliefs and leading to self-reflection as people try to make sense of what has happened. Although it can be distressing, this self-reflection process is directed at rebuilding the individual's beliefs, ideas, and values, eventually leading to PTG.

Seen from this perspective, PTG can be the outcome of the traumatic stress response. Knowing this can provide much needed hope for survivors themselves as they struggle to deal with the challenges of trauma. The following metaphor of the shattered vase is often helpful.

Adversity shakes us to the core because it challenges our beliefs about ourselves and our place in the world. Adversity may show us that we are vulnerable, less important in the grand scheme of things than we thought, or that things we thought to be true just aren't. To overcome adversity and move on, we need to rebuild our belief systems. This can be illustrated through the metaphor of the shattered vase. Imagine that one day you accidentally knock a treasured vase off its perch. It smashes into tiny pieces. What do you do? Do you try to put the vase back together as it was? Like the vase held together by glue and sticky tape, those who try to put their lives back together exactly as they were remain fractured and vulnerable. Or do you pick up the beautiful coloured pieces and use them to make something new—such as a colourful mosaic? Those who accept the breakage and build themselves anew become more resilient and open to new ways of living. The secret to dealing with adversity is to know that you can't put the vase back together exactly as it was, but instead start to use the pieces to build a new mosaic—to find ways in which we can be more true to ourselves, live each day more meaningfully, and work out what really matters to us (see, Joseph 2013).

Conclusion

For those dealing with trauma and losses, understanding that what they are going through has the potential to be a springboard for something positive can be a hopeful message. It can also seem unrealistic and naïve to those in the midst of suffering. This is understandable, but it is our experiences with hundreds of clients who have sought help that although the journey can be long and arduous, it can lead to growth.

One of the most remarkable advances in our knowledge of trauma in recent years is that, in the aftermath of the struggle with adversity, it is common to find benefits. The perception of benefits, in turn, may lead to higher levels of psychological functioning and improved health. This is not to overlook the personal devastation of psychological trauma, but, equally, we must not overlook the fact that psychological trauma does not necessarily lead to a damaged life. Simply being aware of the possibility of benefits can offer hope to people.

References

Affleck, G., Tennen, H., Croog, S., and Levine, S. (1987). Causal attribution, perceived benefits, and morbidity after a heart attack: an 8-year study. *Journal of Consulting and Clinical Psychology* 55, 29–35.

Calhoun, L. G., and Tedeschi, R. G. (2012). *Posttraumatic growth in clinical practice.* London: Routledge.

Helgeson, V. S., Reynolds, K. A., and Tomich, P. L. (2006). A meta-analytic review of benefit finding and growth. *Journal of Consulting and Clinical Psychology* 74(5), 797.

Joseph, S. (2013). *What doesn't kill us: a guide to overcoming adversity and moving forward.* London: Piatkus Little-Brown.

Joseph, S., Maltby, J., Wood, A. M., Stockton, H., Hunt, N., and Regel, S. (2012). The Psychological Well-Being—Post-Traumatic Changes Questionnaire (PWB-PTCQ): reliability and validity. *Psychological Trauma: Theory, Research, Practice, and Policy* 4(4), 420.

Joseph, S., Murphy, D., and Regel, S. (2012). An affective-cognitive processing model of post-traumatic growth. *Clinical Psychology and Psychotherapy* 19, 316–325.

Joseph, S., Williams, R., and Yule, W. (1993). Changes in outlook following disaster: the preliminary development of a measure to assess positive and negative responses. *Journal of Traumatic Stress* 6(2), 271–279.

Linley, P. A., and Joseph, S. (2004). Positive change following trauma and adversity: a review. *Journal of Traumatic Stress* 17(1), 11–21.

Poulin, M. J., Silver, R. C., Gil–Rivas, V., Holman, E. A., and McIntosh, D. N. (2009). Finding social benefits after a collective trauma: perceiving societal changes and well–being following 9/11. *Journal of Traumatic Stress* 22(2), 81–90.

Stanton, A. L., Danoff-Burg S., Sworowski, L. A., Collins, C. A., Branstetter, A. D., Rodriguez-Hanley, A., . . . and Austenfeld, J. L. (2002). Randomized, controlled trial of written emotional expression and benefit finding in breast cancer patients. *Journal of Clinical Oncology* 20(20), 4160–4168.

Tedeschi, R. G., and Calhoun, L. G. (1996). The Posttraumatic Growth Inventory: measuring the positive legacy of trauma. *Journal of Traumatic Stress* 9(3), 455–471.

Woodward, C., and Joseph, S. (2003). Positive change processes and post–traumatic growth in people who have experienced childhood abuse: understanding vehicles of change. *Psychology and Psychotherapy: Theory, Research and Practice* 76(3), 267–283.

11

Self-help

Some things you can do to help yourself or others to promote recovery

---

➔ Key Points

- This chapter aims to offer some thoughts and suggestions that will help to promote recovery and growth following exposure to traumatic events.

- Some of the suggestions will also be helpful to those who have been affected by traumatic bereavement.

- In particular, there is often a need for people to overcome their tendency towards avoidance following trauma and make sure they are engaging with necessary practical and emotional issues.

- Obviously, everyone affected by traumatic events and traumatic bereavement will respond differently, having different emotional resources, levels of natural resilience, and access to social support.

- It is important to try to seek support from those close to you such as family, friends, or colleagues. If this is not possible, then suggestions for more formal support are offered.

Introduction

If you, a loved one, or a friend has recently been through a traumatic event (e.g. a road-traffic collision [RTC]), experienced an assault, or witnessed an accident, say within the past few weeks, and have experienced some or many of what have been described herein as common reactions to such events, there are some helpful things you can do, or help others with, to promote recovery and growth. Avoidance is one of the most common reactions. This is illustrated in Susan's story.

📄 Susan's story

Susan was driving her car on a major motorway during the early evening, returning from work. She was involved in a collision after a car overtook her at speed, colliding with a heavy-goods vehicle, which was behind her. The resulting collision involved her car being spun across the carriageway, facing into the path of oncoming cars. She was not injured but badly shaken and had to be freed by the Fire Service from the car, which took almost 30 minutes. She was taken to hospital but released home in a few hours in the care of her husband. She took 3 days off work, as suggested by her manager, but returned using a courtesy car. Initially she was naturally apprehensive when driving, but this apprehension began to increase gradually in a space of a few days. She soon found that she was taking opportunities to avoid driving on dual carriageways and motorways, and then began avoiding relatively short journeys. She soon started to become apprehensive and anxious even at the thought of driving or being a passenger. Within 4 weeks of the accident, she had almost stopped altogether, and this inevitably affected her work and social life. She would avoid talking about it and started gradually to cut herself off from friends and extended family.

Susan is quite typical in her reactions. Her avoidance and anxiety in the early stages were understandable and what she needed to do because her feelings were so overwhelming. However, over time if she continues to be avoidant and withdrawn from other people, it will almost certainly serve to maintain and worsen her problems.

The key issue for people is to find ways in which to reverse the tendency towards avoidance, to prevent it spiralling out of control and creating further destruction in their lives.

Accessing and accepting support from others

It is very comforting to receive physical and emotional support from other people. It is important not to reject support by trying to appear strong (e.g. demonstrating a 'the stiff upper lip', or trying to cope completely on your own).

Talking with others who have had similar experiences or who understand what you have been through is particularly important. It can allow you to release pent-up feelings and enable barriers to come down and closer relationships to develop.

Some friends may be reluctant to offer their support, even though they would like to help. Often this is because they may not know how to approach you or fear upsetting you by bringing up the subject of what happened. Do not be afraid to ask for and say what you want.

As mentioned in previous chapters, there is overwhelming evidence showing that social support is a major protective factor following exposure to traumatic events or significant life crises. This will also enhance the natural resilience of individuals, families, and communities.

Monitor your reactions over time. The most important consideration is to watch out for any avoidance behaviour, as described earlier. It is often very common for people who have been through a traumatic experience to want to avoid thoughts, places, activities, or people who may remind them in some way of their experience. Given the wide range of traumatic experiences that a person may encounter, this can be an extensive list. However, if this continues, it almost always leads to further problems in the longer term.

Therefore, it is helpful to encourage yourself, or the affected person, to begin gradually to face fearful situations. The simplest way to do this is to try small steps slowly increasing the frequency and duration of the exposure to the feared situation. It is often said that the best way to deal with situations, as in Susan's case above, is 'to get back on the horse'. The important factor here is how one 'gets back on the horse', because it is best to 'get back on the horse' when it is tethered to a post and someone is holding the reins, rather than when it is galloping past! The message is that doing too much too soon can be detrimental, and it can have an aversive effect and lead to further avoidance. Therefore, for example, some simple stages for somebody like Susan, who has been in an RTC, would be to:

♦ Just sit in the car.

♦ Sit in the car with the engine running.

♦ Drive very short distances in familiar settings (e.g. down the street and back).

♦ Increase driving time and distances in familiar settings.

♦ Drive on familiar roads in quiet times.

♦ Drive on familiar roads at busy times.

As can be seen, this could be extended as necessary; however, there are some very simple but important rules that should be followed for exposure to feared situations to be effective: activities should be frequent enough and, above all, there should be consistency.

Taking time out for yourself

In order to deal with their feelings, some people find it necessary at times to be alone or just be with close friends or family. Sometimes this can be difficult when we lead busy lives and have to negotiate carefully with our friends and family to make space for ourselves.

Confronting what has happened

Confronting the reality of the situation (e.g. by talking to a close friend, colleague, or confidante), will help individuals to come to terms with the event. This can be the hardest thing, to accept the reality of our losses and face up to the way in which our life has changed. But although this is important, it's also important to recognize we all have our own ways and speed of doing this, and we should not try to rush people.

Staying active

Helping others, keeping busy, and engaging in previously enjoyed activities can give some temporary relief. Physical activity is really beneficial to our psychological well-being. Research has shown that 30 minutes of activity a day (e.g. walking and gardening) can have a positive effect on mood. So we would recommend strongly that people manage to maintain their activity levels. Often we won't feel like it following trauma, and so it requires that little bit extra effort. It can be simple things, like taking the stairs when you would rather take the lift or walking instead of taking the car. Even if you take exercise in periods of a few minutes, say 10–20 minutes at a time, it is still useful.

Returning to usual and familiar routines

It is usually advisable to return to usual routines as soon as possible after the event in order to avoid incubation and magnification of fear while away from the situation. While it is important to try to return to our routines because of those benefits, people will have different speeds at which they can do this.

New interests

There is also a window of opportunity following trauma to make new changes in life. For example, taking up new activities, interests, and socializing can be helpful to people in the recovery process.

All of the above can prove very helpful and make your experience easier to bear. However, overuse of some coping mechanisms can be counterproductive and even detrimental if they divert you from getting the help and support you need. Overactivity or excessive use of distraction, for example, can be unhelpful if it prevents you confronting the reality of the event. Your recovery may be delayed if you suppress your feelings too much or for too long (numbness), or if you become preoccupied with repeated thoughts of the event. Gradually confronting the reality of what has happened, accepting support from others, and talking through your feelings are particularly important ways of gaining emotional release and coming to terms with your experiences.

Look for post-traumatic growth

As we saw in Chapter 10, often as people begin to recover from trauma, they notice that they have begun to look at life differently. For example, it may be that you find yourself appreciating your friends and family in a new way or you think about what really matters to you in life in a new way or you begin to recognize changes within yourself, such as newfound confidence, maturity, and authenticity. It can be helpful to look actively for such changes in yourself, how you view others, and what matters to you. Begin to notice these changes in yourself. Value the new you and look for ways to do things differently (Joseph, 2013).

Self-acceptance

As we have seen throughout this text, trauma throws up lots of difficult emotions for people. In one way or another, it can be hard to be kind, compassionate, and accepting towards ourselves, thinking we should have acted differently, that we could be coping better, or that we are not good enough. Such feelings and thoughts can get in our way because naturally they make us want to go into hiding and avoid things. We have seen how destructive avoidance can be, so being able to accept ourselves and be kind and compassionate towards ourselves can be very helpful, and it set us on the road to a more growthful recovery. Ask yourself, if it were a loved friend or family member going through what you are going through, would you speak to that person the way you speak to yourself? Would you expect the same things from him or her as you expect from yourself? Be as compassionate to yourself as you would be to others you care about.

Whom should I talk to?

Generally speaking, it is 'good to talk' about our reactions and feelings about what has happened. In the main, it is probably best to talk with people you know, trust, and feel comfortable with—usually this will be with members of your family or with close friends. Sometimes, however, this may not be possible—you may be away from your family and friends, your family or friends may themselves have been involved, or you may find it difficult to talk about your feelings within your family (because you do not wish to upset them or because relationships are strained). If this is the case, you might find it helpful to talk to colleagues at work, to your general practitioner, or a member of the clergy or seek professional mental health advice and support. Remember though that you do not 'have' to talk to a counsellor or therapist if you don't want to, and that, where possible, it is usually enough to draw upon usual forms of support, your family or significant others.

There are different types of counsellor and psychotherapist available. Cognitive-behavioural counsellors and psychotherapists offer structured approaches and focus on identifying the ways in which your thinking affects your behaviours and emotions and how by changing your thinking patterns, you can gradually change how you feel. After the trauma, they are also interested in helping you interpret and understand the 'meaning' of the experience, which for many trauma survivors is a significant factor that can affect the course of their reactions. For example, whilst assessing a young woman who had been a victim of a violent armed robbery at the bank where she worked, she became perplexed by her inability to understand why she was still affected almost 2 years later despite 25 sessions of previous therapy. It transpired that the therapist had focused almost exclusively on the other stressors that were present in her life at the time. Whilst this was also very important, the 'meaning' of the index traumatic experience was not addressed. It transpired that at the time of the robbery, she was saying goodbye to her husband, who had dropped her off at work that day. They were both standing at the door of the bank when the raiders confronted them before running past them and into the bank. When she was describing the event, she became tearful, saying this always happened when she thought about the experience. When asked about her immediate thoughts at the time, she recalled that she was thinking about her children being orphaned if she and her husband had been killed. She reported that she had never been asked about this previously. Cognitive behavioural therapy (CBT) therapists will work collaboratively with you to develop strategies that will help you come to terms with the experience. For example, traumatized people are almost always very avoidant of fearful situations, and so therapists encourage people to confront their experiences, either in imagination, or in real life.

Other types of therapists may also help us to move forwards towards post-traumatic growth or to understand how childhood shaped us as people, and how by helping us make sense of our pasts, we can take more control of our future. Often we become aware of things we weren't previously aware of before. Different therapists will offer different things, but never be scared to ask them about what they are doing. Good therapists will be pleased to explain why they are doing what they are doing.

When to seek professional help

It is important that you allow yourself to talk to your family or friends about your experiences and feelings at the earliest opportunity. If, however, some of the reactions described in Chapter 1 are particularly intense and distressing, or if they persist or have persisted for a long time (for more than about 6 to 8 weeks), it is advisable to seek professional help, sooner rather than later. Some of the pointers that suggest you should consider asking for help include:

♦ If you feel that you are overwhelmed by and cannot handle intense feelings and bodily sensations.

♦ If you have no one to share your emotions with and you feel the need to do so.

♦ You continue to feel numb and empty or have persistent feelings of tension, confusion, exhaustion, or other unpleasant bodily sensations.

♦ You have to keep overactive in order not to focus on your feelings.

♦ You want to avoid thoughts, places, activities, or people who may remind you in some way, however subtle, of your experience.

♦ You continue to have frequent distressing thoughts or recollections of the traumatic experience.

♦ You continue to have nightmares or poor sleep.

♦ Your relationships seem to be suffering badly or sexual problems develop.

♦ You find that you are drinking to excess.

♦ Your work performance suffers, you make mistakes, or you have accidents associated with poor concentration.

It may be helpful to try the Trauma-Screening Questionnaire (TSQ), which is a self-report scale of individual responses to a traumatic event (Box. 11.1). It consists of ten questions measuring re-experiencing of the event and symptoms of arousal. It is designed for use a month or more following exposure to a traumatic event (it is not designed to be used before that time), to identify individuals who may be suffering from symptoms of post-traumatic stress. It only takes a few minutes to complete, and the scoring is simple and straightforward. It assesses current symptoms and does not diagnose post-traumatic stress disorder (PTSD). It is based on research conducted with train crash survivors. Answering yes, to six or more items could mean that the person may be at risk of suffering from the early stages of PTSD and would benefit from further detailed assessment.

Other important points to remember

If you have experienced a personal loss as a result of the incident, then the time taken to process and come to terms with the loss may take considerably longer (e.g. months and sometimes years; see Chapter 4 on traumatic bereavement).

In addition, changes in outlook and attitude towards others and the world are common; these may be lasting and will fluctuate over time, but in most cases, they are for the better, and the effects are positive. However, if they are

> **Box 11.1** The Trauma-Screening Questionnaire (TSQ)
>
> **Your own reactions now to the traumatic event**
>
> Please consider the following reactions which sometimes occur after a traumatic event. This questionnaire is concerned with your personal reactions to the traumatic event which happened to you. Please indicate (Yes/No) whether or not you have experienced any of the following at least twice in the past week.
>
> 1. Upsetting thoughts or memories about the event that have come into your mind against your will
>
> 2. Upsetting dreams about the event
>
> 3. Acting or feeling as though the event were happening again
>
> 4. Feeling upset by reminders of the event
>
> 5. Bodily reactions (such as fast heartbeat, stomach churning, sweatiness, dizziness) when reminded of the event
>
> 6. Difficulty falling or staying asleep
>
> 7. Irritability or outbursts of anger
>
> 8. Difficulty concentrating
>
> 9. Heightened awareness of potential dangers to yourself and others
>
> 10. Being jumpy or being startled at something unexpected
>

becoming problematic, confusing, or distressing, they can be addressed with professional help.

Anniversaries will be coming up, as will birthdays and other memorable occasions. Whilst these will be distressing, try to commemorate them in your own way. Inevitably, there may be family tensions and disagreements (This is very normal!), aim for compromise and agree to differ. If need be, hold separate small personal ceremonies.

Some dos and don'ts to remember

DO

◆ Express your emotions, take the opportunity to review the experience within yourself and with others and let your family share in your experiences.

◆ Express your needs clearly and honestly to your family and friends and your managers and colleagues at work.

◆ Take time out to sleep, rest, think, and be with your close family and friends.

◆ Try to keep your life as normal as possible after the initial period of often intense acute distress.

DON'T

◆ Bottle up feelings, avoid talking about what has happened, or let your embarrassment stop you giving others the chance to talk.

◆ Expect the memories to go away quickly—they may stay with you for some time.

◆ Forget that if others are involved—they may be experiencing similar feelings to yours.

Whilst people often say that after a traumatic event, 'Things will never be the same again …', to some extent this may be true, but do remember that you are basically the same person that you were before the incident and that if you feel unable to cope with your feelings and reactions, support and advice is available.

Where to seek professional help

If you wish to find out more about the availability of confidential counselling, in the first instance, you should, approach your own GP or family doctor, who will be able to advise you on the options available in your area and put you in touch with someone who can help. This may be:

◆ A counsellor in the doctor's surgery.

◆ A mental health professional from the local community mental health team or services (psychiatrist community mental health nurse, social worker, psychologist, specialist therapist, or occupational therapist).

◆ Some areas have specialist trauma and bereavement services and, again, these can be accessed by your doctor. Some accept self-referrals, so it is often worth contacting them for more information.

◆ Currently, in many regions of England, there is a service—Improving Access to Psychological Therapies (IAPT). It was created to offer individuals realistic, routine first-line 'talking therapies', combined, where appropriate, with medication, which traditionally had been the only treatment available. Family doctors can refer to IAPT and the service also accepts self-referrals for the lower-level interventions, usually 6–8 sessions.

◆ If there are no specialist services locally, in the UK, your family doctor can apply to the local Clinical Commissioning Group, who can fund you to attend specialist services for assessment and treatment in a neighbouring county or another part of the country.

◆ Other options are to seek support from organizations such as Cruse Bereavement Care and Victim Support. There is a list at the end of the book. In other countries, this will differ and, in some cases, it may be provided by organizations such as the Red Cross National Society. In the case of traumatic bereavement resulting from homicide in the UK, there is the Victim Support (VS) National Homicide Service. In the first instance, a police officer, usually known as a Family Liaison Officer, will ask the individual or family if they wish to have a VS homicide service caseworker assigned to their case. The caseworkers are experienced professionals and have been specifically trained to provide a range of practical support interventions, including signposting individuals for specialist psychological help if needed.

◆ You may wish to seek help privately from a therapist or counsellor. Don't hesitate to ask them about their experience, qualifications, and, most importantly, their experience of working with psychological trauma or traumatic bereavement. This is especially important if you are seeing them in the early stages after experiencing an event; say within the first 4–12 weeks. Also if you are seen within that time frame, ensure you are offered a follow-up appointment. In addition, if you decide to pursue this as an avenue of help, it is important to find someone with whom you feel comfortable and safe.

Conclusion

Deciding whether an individual is experiencing problems or a range of reactions that will spontaneously resolve after a traumatic event can be difficult. Understanding and being aware of the psychological trajectory of the response within the first 6–8 weeks can be helpful in determining the probable course of the person's reactions. If the initial distress is steadily diminishing in frequency, intensity, and duration, then there is every chance that recovery and a return to what for that person would be stability and equilibrium. However, if the reactions persist or are increasingly problematic, advice, guidance, and support should be sought. Remember that following traumatic bereavement, the time frame will be considerably longer. A mental health assessment may be appropriate to assess and determine individual needs, with attention being paid to a risk assessment and other factors, such as previous vulnerabilities and social support. Information from relatives can also be an important part of this process. Interventions that include education, advice, and guidance, based on and related to the person's unique experience, can be helpful. Follow-up is important to assess progress over the following months.

References

Brewin, C. et al. (2002). Brief screening instrument for post-traumatic stress disorder. *British Journal of Psychiatry* **181**, 158–162.

Joseph, S. (2013). *What doesn't kill us: a guide to overcoming adversity and moving forward.* London: Piatkus.

Appendix 1

Further Reading

General

Brewin, C. R. (2003). *Post-traumatic stress disorder: malady or myth?* New Haven and London: Yale University Press. A very readable overview of the nature of trauma and some of the critiques surrounding PTSD.

Cash, A. (2006). *Posttraumatic stress disorder. Wiley concise guides to mental health.* Hoboken: Wiley. A good introductory textbook to the field that discusses different theories and therapeutic approaches.

Beck, J.G., and Sloan, D.M (2012) The Oxford Handbook of Traumatic Stress Disorders. New York. Oxford University Press. A through and comprehensive text on trauma and PTSD primarily for academics and researchers.

Herman, J. L. (1992). *Trauma and recovery—from domestic abuse to physical terror.* London: Harper Collins. Seen by many as a seminal work. For general readership (as well as professional), a historical and political overview of trauma and explorations of gender and trauma.

van der Kolk, B. A., McFarlane, A. C., and Weisaeth, L., eds. (1996). *Traumatic stress.* New York: Guilford. Remains a thorough and comprehensive textbook on all aspects of trauma and PTSD with contributions from leading researchers in the field.

Post-traumatic growth

Calhoun, L. G., and Tedeschi, R. G. (2012). *Posttraumatic growth in clinical practice.* London: Routledge. Informative guide for therapists to understand and help to facilitate PTG.

Joseph, S., and Linley, P. A., eds. (2008). *Trauma, recovery, and growth: positive psychological perspectives on post-traumatic stress.* Hoboken: Wiley. Especially useful to professionals who want to know more about research and findings about PTG in different contexts, such as cancer, terrorism, and combat.

Psycho-social management of disasters

Gibson, M. (2006). *Order from chaos: responding to traumatic events.* 3rd ed. Birmingham: Policy Press. A very readable and practical text about the impact and management of disasters, especially for those responding in the emergency phases.

International Federation of Red Cross and Red Crescent Societies. (published annually). *World disasters report*. Oxford: Oxford University Press. A good overview of disasters and the international responses, usually with different themes. Useful for statistics.

Ursano, R. J., McCaughy, B., and Fullerton, C., eds. (1994). *Individual and community responses to disaster*. Cambridge: Cambridge University Press. A comprehensive textbook on disasters and their aftermath.

Working with trauma in different cultural contexts

Marsella, A. J., Freidman, M. J., Gerrity, E. T., and Scurfield, R., eds. (1996). *Ethnocultural Aspects of post-traumatic stress disorder—issues, research and clinical applications*. Washington, DC: American Psychiatric Press. A very comprehensive textbook on trauma in different cultural contexts.

Schauer, M., Neuner, F., and Elbert, T. (2011). *Narrative exposure therapy: a short-term intervention for traumatic stress disorders after war, terror or torture*. Washington, DC: Hogrefe & Huber. An excellent overview of the theory and application Narrative Exposure Therapy (NET).

Van der Veer, G. (1992). *Counselling and therapy with refugees—psychological problems of victims of war, torture and repression*. New York: Wiley. A useful and practical text on counselling with refugee populations.

Wilson, J. P., and Drozdek, B., eds. (2004). *Broken spirits: the treatment of traumatized asylum seekers, refugees, war and torture victims*. New York: Brunner-Routledge. A comprehensive textbook on approaches to working with the populations referred to in the title.

Treatment

Follette, V., and Ruzek, J., eds. (2006). Cognitive-behavioural therapies for trauma. 2nd ed. London: Guilford Press. Some useful chapters, especially an excellent chapter on working with trauma-related guilt.

Jehu, D. (1988). *Beyond sexual abuse—cognitive therapy with women who were childhood victims*. New York: Wiley. Not new, but a good text on understanding how cognitive therapy can be effective with survivors of sexual abuse, with many clinical examples.

Shapiro, F., and Forrest, M. S. (1997). *EMDR: the breakthrough therapy for overcoming anxiety, stress and trauma*. New York: Basic Books. A general introduction on EMDR, suitable for the professional and the more-informed lay reader.

Yule, W., ed. (2003). *Post-traumatic stress disorders: concepts and therapy*. 3rd ed. Chichester: Wiley. An excellent overview of concepts such as social support and attribution and their role in the spectrum of trauma responses.

Trauma and children

Dyregrov, A. (2008). *Grief in young children: a handbook for adults*. London: Jessica Kingsley.

Dyregrov, A. (2010). *Supporting traumatised children and teenagers: a guide to providing understanding and help*. London: Jessica Kingsley. Excellent for understanding the responses of children and teenagers to trauma loss and grief, and very readable and practical.

Harris-Hendriks, J., Black, D., and Kaplan, T. (2000). *When father kills mother—guiding children through trauma and grief*. 2nd ed. London: Routledge. A very good guide for those working with children and families affected by sudden traumatic bereavement following homicide.

Yule, W., and Gold, A. (1993). *Wise before the event: coping with crises in schools*. London: Calouste Gulbenkian Foundation. For teachers and others—an excellent guide to preparing for and coping with crises in educational settings.

Trauma in the workplace

Australian Centre for Posttraumatic Mental Health. (2011). Development of guidelines on peer support using the Delphi methodology. *ACPMH*. (www.acpmh.unimelb.edu.au). Useful recommendations for peer support initiatives in organizations.

The British Psychological Society. (2002). *Psychological debriefing: professional practice board working party*. Leicester: BPS. The BPS's report on psychological debriefing, which can be found online at the BPS website (http://www.bps.org.uk/).

Dyregov, A. (2003). *Psychological debriefing: a leader's guide for small group crisis intervention*. Ellicott City: Chevron Publishing Corporation. The best practical guide to the subject of group crisis intervention and debriefing.

Everley, G. S., and Mitchell, J. T. (2008). *Integrative crisis intervention and disaster mental health*. Ellicott City, MD: Chevron Publishing. A general overview of Critical Incident Stress Management and Critical Incident Stress. Debriefing; useful for the emergency services.

Hughes, R., Kinder, A., and Cooper, C., eds. (2012). *International handbook of workplace trauma support*. London: Wiley-Blackwell. A recent and comprehensive overview of theory and practice in the field of workplace trauma support.

Raphael, B., and Wilson, J. P., eds. (2000). *Psychological debriefing: theory, practice and evidence*. Cambridge: Cambridge University Press. An academic textbook devoted to the research and practice in the area, with chapters by detractors and supporters of CISM and PD.

Culture/societies in conflict

Smyth, M., and Fay, M-T. (2000). *Personal accounts from Northern Ireland's Troubles*. London: Pluto

Personal stories and testimonies from those affected by the Troubles. (1999). *Truth and Reconciliation Commission of South Africa Report*. Vols. 1–5. 2nd ed. London: MacMillan. Comprehensive and moving testimonies and accounts from the TRC proceedings. A fascinating insight into a country trying to come to terms with its past.

Bereavement and grief

De Leo, D., Cimitan, A., and Dyregrov, K., eds., (2013). *Bereavement after sudden death: helping the survivors*. Gottingen: Hogrefe. Another very useful guide for practitioners.

Dyregrov, K., and Dyregrov, A. (2008). *Effective grief and bereavement support*. London: Jessica Kingsley. Does exactly what it says in the title; very practical, with lots of suggestions for intervening in different contexts and settings.

Pearlman, L. A., Wortman, C. B., Feuer, C. A., and Farber, C. H. (2014). *Treating traumatic bereavement: a practitioner's guide*. New York: Guilford. A useful guide for practitioners wanting to increase the therapeutic repertoire.

Stroebe, M. S., Hansson, R.O., Schut, H., and Stroebe, W. (2008). *Handbook of bereavement research and practice: advances in theory and intervention*. Washington, DC: APA. This is a comprehensive overview of research and practice in bereavement and loss.

Trauma and the law

Napier, M., and Wheat, K. (2005). *Recovering damages for psychiatric injury*. 2nd ed. Oxford: Oxford University Press. A comprehensive overview and guide to the law in relation to psychiatric injury and employer's liability, and duty of care, for example; essential reading for solicitors and those preparing psychiatric reports.

Self-help guides

These books may be helpful where other problems are present in addition to PTSD or related to the development and maintenance of the problem (e.g. obsessive-compulsive disorder). They are accessible and practical and can be used as an adjunct to therapy by the therapist and patient.

De Silva, P., and Rachman, S. (2009). *Obsessive compulsive disorder: the facts*. 4th ed. Oxford: Oxford University Press.

Fennell, M. (2009). *Overcoming low self-esteem: a self-help guide using cognitive behavioural techniques*. London: Robinson.

Gilbert, P. (2009). *Overcoming depression: a self-help guide using cognitive behavioural techniques*. 2nd ed. London: Robinson.

Joseph, S. (2013). *What doesn't kill us: a guide to overcoming adversity and moving forward*. London: Piatkus Little-Brown.

Kennerley, H. (2000). *Overcoming Childhood trauma: a self-help guide using cognitive behavioural techniques*. London: Robinson.

Moncrieff, J. (2009). *A straight talking introduction to psychiatric drugs*. Ross on Wye: PCCS Books.

Silove, D., and Manicavasagar, V. (2009). *Overcoming panic and agoraphobia: a self-help guide using cognitive behavioural techniques*. London: Robinson.

Appendix 2

Useful websites

Aberdeen Centre for Trauma Research, Robert Gordon University, Aberdeen
http://www.rgu.ac.uk/actr/general/page.cfm

American Journal of Psychiatry
http://ajp.psychiatryonline.org/

American Psychological Association
http://www.apa.org/

Amnesty International
http://www.amnesty.org.uk/

Anxiety UK
http://www.anxietyuk.org.uk/

Australasian Society for Traumatic Stress Studies
http://www.astss.org.au/

Australian Psychological Society
http://www.psychsociety.org.au

Brake: The road's charity
http://www.brake.org.uk/

British Association for Behavioural and Cognitive Psychotherapies
http://www.babcp.com/Default.aspx

British Journal of Psychiatry
http://bjp.rcpsych.org/

British Psychological Society
http://www.bps.org.uk/

British Red Cross
http://www.redcross.org.uk/

Canadian Psychiatric Association
http://www.cpa-apc.org/

Canadian Psychological Association
http://www.cpa.ca/

Centre for Crisis Psychology, Bergen, Norway
http://www.krisepsyk.no/

Centre for Trauma Resilience and Growth, Nottingham, UK
http://www.nottinghamshirehealthcare.nhs.uk/trauma

Children and War
http://www.childrenandwar.org/

Combat Stress
http://www.combatstress.org.uk/

Cruse Bereavement Care
http://www.crusebereavementcare.org.uk/

David Baldwin's Trauma Pages
An excellent portal for trauma related information and resources
http://www.trauma-pages.com/

Department of Health—Improving Access to Psychological Therapies
http://www.iapt.nhs.uk/

Disaster Action
http://www.disasteraction.org.uk/

Escaping Victimhood
The website provides excellent information for employers supporting those traumatically bereaved through homicide or other traumatic loss.
http://www.escapingvictimhood.com/

Forced Migration Online
http://www.forcedmigration.org

Harvard Program in Refugee Trauma
http://hprt-cambridge.org/

Hostage UK
Hostage UK is an independent charity that supports hostages and their families during and after an overseas kidnap. They also work with various related organizations to improve their family response and conduct research to enhance public understanding. In 2016, Hostage established a US base in partnership with the James W Foley Legacy Foundation.
http://www.hostageuk.org

Human Rights Watch
http://www.hrw.org

International Committee of the Red Cross (ICRC)
The ICRC is an independent, neutral organization ensuring humanitarian protection and assistance for victims of war and other situations of violence.
http://www.icrc.org

International Crisis Incident Stress Foundation
http://www.icisf.org

International Federation of Red Cross and Red Crescent Societies
http://www.ifrc.org/

International Federation of Red Cross and Red Crescent Societies Reference Centre for Psychosocial Support
http://psp.drk.dk/sw2955.asp

International Rehabilitation Centre for Torture Victims
http://www.irct.org

International Society for Traumatic Stress Studies
http://www.istss.org

Medecins Sans Frontieres
http://www.msf.org/

Medical Foundation for the Care of Victims of Torture
http://www.torturecare.org.uk

National Centre for PTSD Washington (and for PILOTS database)
http://www.ncptsd.org/

National Institute for Clinical Excellence
http://www.nice.org.uk/

NICE Guidelines PTSD link
http://guidance.nice.org.uk/CG26

Refugee Studies Centre, University of Oxford
http://www.rsc.ox.ac.uk

South African Institute for Traumatic Stress
http://www.saits.org.za/

The European Society for Traumatic Stress
http://www.estss.org/

The Inter-Agency Standing Committee
This is the primary mechanism for interagency coordination of humanitarian assistance involving the key UN and non-UN humanitarian partners.
http://humanitarianonfo/org/iasc

UK Psychological Trauma Society
http://www.ukpts.co.uk

UK Resilience
http://www.cabinetoffice.gov.uk/ukresilience.aspx

UK Trauma Group
The website offers resources in the UK for accessing treatment in local areas.
http://www.uktrauma.org.uk/

United Nations High Commissioner for Refugees

http://www.unhcr.org

Victim Support

http://www.victimsupport.org.uk

VIVO Foundation (For Narrative Exposure Therapy—NET)

http://www.vivo.org/

Index